Clinical Data Interpretation for Medical Finals

Single Best Answer Questions

Clinical Data Interpretation for Medical Finals

Single Best Answer Questions

Edited by

Mr Philip Socrates Pastides
MBBS BSc(Hons) MAcadMEd MRCS(Eng)
Core Surgical Trainee, Royal National Orthopaedic Hospital NHS Trust, Stanmore, London, UK

Ms Parveen Jayia
MBBS MRCS(Eng) MRPharmS(Hons)
Core Surgical Trainee, St Mary's Hospital, Imperial College Healthcare NHS Trust, London, UK

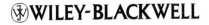

A John Wiley & Sons, Ltd., Publication

This edition first published 2012 © 2012 by Philip Socrates Pastides and Parveen Jayia

Wiley-Blackwell is an imprint of John Wiley & Sons, formed by the merger of Wiley's global Scientific, Technical and Medical business with Blackwell Publishing.

Registered office: John Wiley & Sons, Ltd, The Atrium, Southern Gate, Chichester, West Sussex, PO19 8SQ, UK

Editorial offices: 9600 Garsington Road, Oxford, OX4 2DQ, UK
                      The Atrium, Southern Gate, Chichester, West Sussex, PO19 8SQ, UK
                      111 River Street, Hoboken, NJ 07030-5774, USA

For details of our global editorial offices, for customer services and for information about how to apply for permission to reuse the copyright material in this book please see our website at www.wiley.com/wiley-blackwell.

Library of Congress Cataloging-in-Publication Data

Clinical data interpretation for medical finals : single best answer questions / edited by Philip Socrates Pastides, Parveen Jayia.
     p. ; cm.
  ISBN 978-0-470-65988-5 (pbk.)
  I. Pastides, Philip Socrates.   II. Jayia, Parveen.
  [DNLM: 1. Clinical Medicine–Examination Questions. WB 18.2]
  616.0076–dc23
                                        2011037227

A catalogue record for this book is available from the British Library.

Wiley also publishes its books in a variety of electronic formats. Some content that appears in print may not be available in electronic books.

Set in 9/12pt Frutiger-Light by Thomson Digital, Noida, India
Printed and bound in Malaysia by Vivar Printing Sdn Bhd

1   2012

Contents

Contributors

Sandeep Basavarajaiah, MBBS MRCP MD, Specialist Registrar in Cardiology, Papworth Hospital, Cambridge, UK

Santino Jacob Capocci, BMedSCI(Hons) BMBS MRCP(Resp) DTM&H, Specialist Registrar in Respiratory Medicine, Royal Free Hospital, London, UK

Claudia Carmaciu, MBBS BSc(Hons), Foundation Year Two, Queens Hospital Romford, London, UK

Neil Chauhan, MBBS MRCP, Specialist Registrar in Haematology, Royal London Hospital, London, UK

Hugo Donaldson, MB BCh MRCP FRCPath, Consultant Microbiologist, Charing Cross Hospital, London, UK

Petrut Gogalniceanu, MBBS BSc MRCS, Specialist Registrar General Surgery, London Postgraduate School of Surgery, London, UK

Parminder Johal, MBBS MD FRCS Ed(Tr&Orth), Consultant Trauma & Orthopaedic Surgeon, North Middlesex Hospital, London, UK

Saleem Khoyratty, MA (Cantab) MBBS, Anaesthetic Senior House Officer, Kent, Surrey, Sussex Deanery

Rohaj Mehta, MBBS MRCP, Consultant Dermatologist, Basildon University Hospital, Essex, UK

Michel Michaelides, BSc MBBS MD FRCOphth, Clinical Senior Lecturer & Consultant Ophthalmologist, UCL Institute of Ophthalmology & Moorfields Eye Hospital, London, UK

Nick Manickam Muthiah, MBBS MEd MRCOphth, Vitreo-Retinal Surgery Clinical Research Fellow, Moorfields Eye Hospital & Institute of Ophthalmology, UCL, London, UK

Paraskevas A Paraskeva, PhD FCRS, Reader in Surgery and Consultant Surgeon, Imperial College London, & Imperial College Healthcare NHS Trust, London, UK

Prasanna Lionel Perera, MBBS MRCP FRCR, Consultant Radiologist, Worthing Hospital, West Sussex, UK

Vimal Raj, MBBS FRCR PGDMLS EDM, Consultant Radiologist, Glenfield Hospital, Leicester, UK

Foreword

It has become almost universal that multi-option questioning forms the mainstay of many of the written components of medical exams. As these have evolved we have seen a change from traditional multiple choice questions with negative marking and black-and-white answers to more scenario-based questions. One of the most popular modern formats is the single-best-answer style, which this book adopts. When written carefully, single best answers can challenge the students' range of abilities and can use more realistic clinical examples.

This book provides advice on exam questions and allows students to test their knowledge with a more modern style of single-best-answer questions, which are based more around clinical situations that would be faced by students, foundation year doctors and junior trainees. All of the questions have full explanatory answers which allow students to learn as they test themselves. There are many question books available, but this one is written to be informative and challenging while ensuring that the foundations of medical and surgical practice are covered and that it is enjoyable to use.

Mr P Paraskeva PhD FRCS
Reader in Surgery Imperial College London

Preface

The idea for this book came to us whilst we were immersed in the final stages of revision for medical school finals. The format for final MBBS had just changed to single best answers, which sounds similar to multiple choice questions, but the two are very different. We soon realised that we had to approach these questions from a different angle.

There are numerous books and teaching materials available for clinical OSCES, MCQs, and EMQs but few that focus purely on clinical data analysis.

In the world of 21st-century medicine, clinicians have access to a large armoury of investigations, from simple blood results to complex imaging. Students should become confident in the analytical interpretation of commonly requested investigations early on in their career. If we cannot analyse the data appropriately we are failing not only our patients but also ourselves as clinicians.

The aim of this book is to arm readers with the skills to be successful in medical examinations and, importantly, to allow them to gain confidence when faced with raw data. The subjects covered focus on aspects of medicine that all clinicians will encounter in their daily practice. We highlight areas that may pose some difficulty in understanding or may have been sidelined during medical training.

We hope you enjoy the book as much we have enjoyed compiling it.

2011
P S Pastides & P Jayia
London, UK

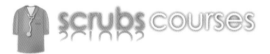

Established in 2007, the principle aim of Scrubscourses is to enhance both undergraduate and post graduate medical education. We offer high quality specialist delivered lecture based and OSCE style courses for all levels.

The courses are well received and unique in that specialists in their field teach all courses.

For more information please visit our website www.scrubscourses.com

We look forward to welcoming you on our future courses.

PSP & PJ

Acknowledgements

My gratitude goes out to all the contributors to this book and the staff at Wiley-Blackwell, without whom none of this would have been possible. Special thanks to my parents, Paul and Nina, my sister Alice and of course my other half, Claudia, who not only contributed to this book, but was forced to take up knitting whilst I spent months putting it together. Last but not least, thank you Parveen for putting up with me!

PSP

I am deeply grateful to my friends, family, the contributors to the book and the staff at Wiley-Blackwell who have supported Philip and me in this adventure. In particular, I would like to thank my parents, Rajinder and Surrinder, and my husband Nick for the comforting shoulder they have provided me. I am sure they will be happy that they will no longer need to listen to my constant grumblings. Finally thank you Philip for agreeing to join me in this adventure. One of many....

PJ

We also warmly acknowledge Mr Salman Rana for assistance with the General Surgery and Gastroenterology chapter and Basildon Medical Photography Department for their assistance with the Dermatology chapter.

Reference Values

Full blood count

Hb	11.5–16.5 g/dL
White cell count (WCC)	$3.8–11.8 \times 10^9$/L
Neutrophils	$2.00–6.77 \times 10^9$/L
Lymphocytes	$1–4 \times 10^9$/L
Monocytes	$0.2–0.8 \times 10^9$/L
Eosinophils	$0.04–0.40 \times 10^9$/L
Basophils	$0.01–0.10 \times 10^9$/L
Platelets	$150–400 \times 10^9$/L
Haematocrit	0.37–0.50 L/L
Mean cell volume (MCV)	78–100 fL

Urea and electrolytes

Sodium	135–145 mmol/L
Potassium	3.5–5.1 mmol/L
Urea	3–8 mmol/L
Creatinine	60–125 mmol/L

Haematinics

Serum iron	11.5–16.5 g/dL
Total iron-binding capacity	250–370 µg/dL
Serum ferritin	20–250 µg/L

Liver profile

Alkaline phosphatase (ALP)	30–150 IU/L
Aspartate transaminase (AST)	3–35 IU/L
Alanine aminotransferase (ALT)	3–35 IU/L
Lactate dehydrogenase	70–250 IU/L
Bilirubin	3–17 µmol/L
Calcium	2.12–2.65 mmol/L
Albumin	35–50 g/L

Clotting profile

Prothrombin time	12–15 s
APTT	28–38 s
Thrombin time	12–15 s
Factor VIIIC	>0.006 IU/mL
Factor vWF	>1.00 IU/mL
D-dimers	<0.25 mg/L

Inflammatory markers

C-reactive protein (CRP)	<8 mg/L
Erythrocyte sedimentation rate (ESR)	<2 mm/hour

Arterial blood gas

pH	7.35–7.45
PaO_2 on air	>10.6 kPa
$PaCO_2$ on air	4.7–6.0 kPa
HCO_3	22–26 mEq/L
Base excess	±2 mmol/L
Lactate	<1.5 mmol/L

1 Cardiac Medicine

Questions

Sandeep Basavarajaiah

Question 1

A 70-year-old Caucasian man with a known history of hypertension, type 2 diabetes mellitus and hypercholesterolaemia presents to A&E with a 2-hour history of central crushing chest pain. His 12-lead ECG performed in A&E is shown below:

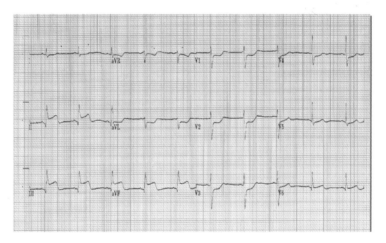

1. What is the diagnosis?

A. Anterior myocardial infarction
B. Inferior myocardial infarction
C. Anterolateral myocardial infarction
D. Acute pericarditis
E. Aortic dissection

Clinical Data Interpretation for Medical Finals: Single Best Answer Questions, First Edition.
Edited by Philip Socrates Pastides and Parveen Jayia.
© 2012 Philip Socrates Pastides and Parveen Jayia. Published 2012 by John Wiley & Sons, Ltd.

2. What is the most appropriate treatment of his condition?
A. Thrombolysis
B. Primary angioplasty
C. Rescue angioplasty
D. Conservative treatment
E. Heparin infusion

Question 2

*A 90-year-old woman is admitted under the general physicians with symp-
toms of recurrent episodes of syncope. She has no significant past medical
history of note except for arthritis, for which she is taking regular paracetamol.
On examination her pulse rate is 40 beats/min and her blood pressure (BP) is
120/80 mmHg. Cardiovascular examination is unremarkable and the 12-lead
ECG performed during her admission is shown below:*

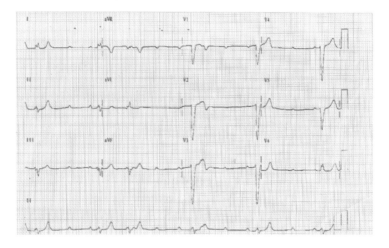

**1. What is your diagnosis based on her ECG and presenting
symptoms?**
A. Sinus bradycardia
B. First-degree heart block
C. Mobitz type 1 atrioventricular (AV) block
D. Mobitz type 2 AV block
E. Complete AV block

2. What is the definitive management of her condition?

A. Atropine

B. Isoprenaline

C. Permanent pacemaker

D. Temporary pacemaker

E. No treatment required

Question 3

A 40-year-old heavy smoker is brought in by the ambulance crew with symptoms of left-sided chest tightness that radiates down his left arm. He is quite unwell in A&E with respiratory distress and sweating. His BP is 120/70 mmHg. Cardiovascular examination reveals normal heart sounds and his 12-lead ECG taken in the department is shown below:

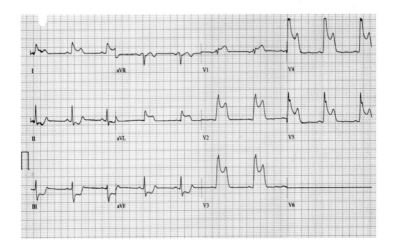

1. What is the diagnosis?

A. Unstable angina

B. Anterolateral myocardial infarction

C. Posterior-myocardial infarction

D. Inferior myocardial infarction

E. Acute pericarditis

2. He subsequently undergoes chest X-ray, the result of which is shown below. What is the diagnosis?

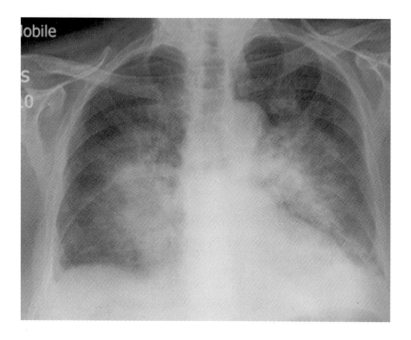

A. Pneumonia
B. Pneumothorax
C. Pulmonary oedema
D. Pericaridal effusion
E. The chest X-ray is normal

Question 4

A 50-year-old man who was previously fit and well was found collapsed at his home by his son. On arrival at A&E he is tachycardic (120 beats/min), hypotensive (systolic BP=80 mmHg), tachypnoeic (respiratory rate of 30/min) and complains of central chest pain. He is saturating at 86% on high-flow oxygen via rebreathable mask. His arterial blood gas (PO2) during admission is 6.1 kPa with metabolic acidosis. His chest X-ray and 12-lead ECG provide an important clue in relation to the diagnosis of his condition and are shown:

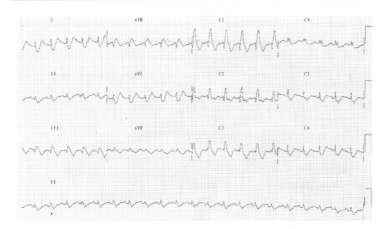

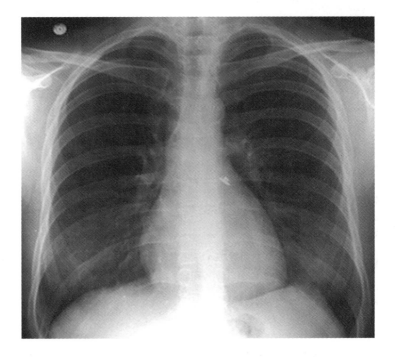

1. What are the two striking abnormalities noted on his ECG?

A. Left bundle branch block
B. Right bundle branch block
C. Atrial fibrillation
D. Supraventricular tachycardia
E. Sinus tachycardia

2. Considering his presentation and clinical picture, what is the underlying diagnosis?

A. Acute myocardial infarction
B. Aortic dissection
C. Acute pulmonary embolism
D. Myocarditis
E. Chronic pulmonary embolism

Question 5

A 54-year-old man who is known to have ischaemic heart disease with two previous myocardial infarctions presents to A&E with a 2-hour history of palpitations. On examination he appears extremely unwell. He is sweating and his systolic BP is 70 mmHg. His 12-lead ECG (below) is diagnostic of his presentation.

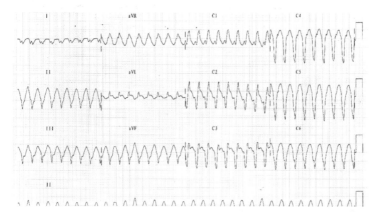

1. What is the diagnosis?

A. Atrial fibrillation

B. AV nodal re-entry tachycardia

C. Ventricular tachycardia

D. Sinus tachycardia

E. Ventricular fibrillation

2. What would be your immediate management of his condition?

A. IV amiodarone

B. IV beta-blocker

C. IV flecainide

D. Emergency cardioversion

E. No treatment required, just observation in the coronary care unit (CCU)

Question 6

A 78-year-old independent woman with a known history of long-standing treated hypertension and type-2 diabetes mellitus complains of 3-day history of shortness of breath and palpitations. A 12-lead ECG carried out at the GP surgery is shown below. On examination her heart rate is 180 beats/min with a BP of 140/70 mmHg. Cardiac auscultation reveals no cardiac murmur.

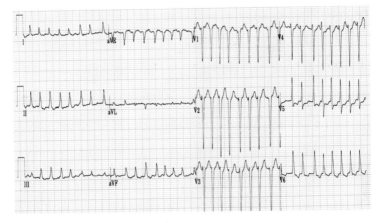

1. What is the diagnosis?

A. Sinus tachycardia

B. Atrial fibrillation

C. Ventricular tachycardia

D. Ventricular fibrillation

E. Atrial tachycardia

2. As per the published National Institute for Health and Clinical Excellence (NICE) guidelines, what would be the first agent of choice in controlling her heart rate?
A. Digoxin
B. Beta-blocker
C. Calcium channel blocker
D. Amiodarone
E. Flecanide

3. What other drug is essential for this patient?
A. Calcium channel blockers
B. Aspirin
C. Warfarin
D. Clopidogrel
E. Digoxin

Question 7

A 35-year-old man with a family history of sudden cardiac death is admitted to A&E with symptoms of palpitations. He is haemodynamically stable with his systolic BP > 100 mmHg. However, his 12-lead ECG (below) is abnormal.

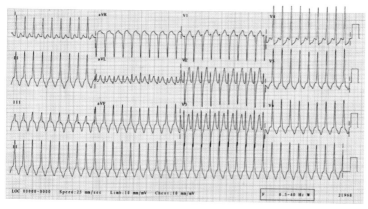

1. What does the ECG show?
A. Supraventricular tachycardia
B. Ventricular tachycardia
C. Sinus tachycardia
D. Atrial fibrillation
E. Ventricular fibrillation

He is subsequently given 12 mg of IV adenosine, which cardioverts him to sinus rhythm and his ECG post-cardioversion is shown below:

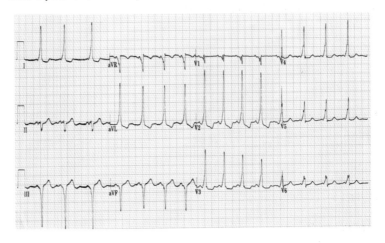

2. What is the diagnosis?

A. Wolff–Parkinson–White (WPW) syndrome

B. Long QT syndrome

C. Left ventricular hypertrophy

D. Left bundle branch block

E. Lown–Ganong–Levine syndrome

3. What will be the definitive management of his condition?

A. Amiodarone

B. Permanent pacemaker insertion

C. Radiofrequency ablation

D. No treatment required

E. Flecanide

Question 8

A 16-year-old girl with congenital bilateral deafness is referred by her GP with symptoms of recurrent palpitations. On two occasions her palpitations have resulted in syncope. One year ago her maternal aunt died suddenly in her sleep, but post-mortem examination failed to shown any pathology. The girl underwent 12-lead ECG at her GP surgery, the result of which is shown:

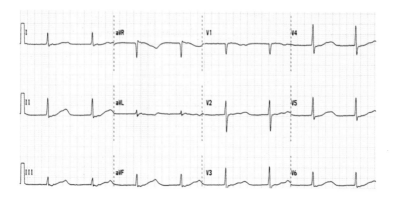

What intervention should this young girl undergo?

A. Radiofrequency ablation
B. Biventricular pacemaker
C. Coronary angiography
D. Intracardiac defibrillator
E. Pulmonary venous isolation

Question 9

An 80-year-old woman presents to A&E with symptoms of recurrent falls. She is a known hypertensive, but her BP has been well controlled with bendrofluazide. Her only other past medical history is hypothyroidism and a recent thyroid function test performed by her GP was within the normal limits. On examination she is normotensive and her heart rate is 64 beats/min. Cardiovascular examination reveals normal heart sounds. Her admission ECG is shown:

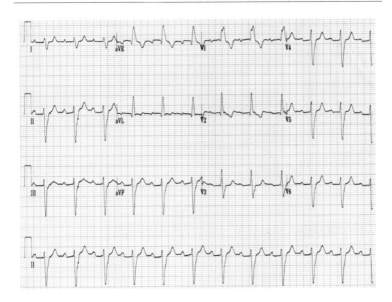

1. What is your diagnosis on the basis of her ECG and presenting symptoms?

A. First-degree AV block
B. Complete AV block
C. Trifascicular block
D. Bifascicular block
E. Unifascicular block

2. What is the definitive management of her condition?

A. Atropine
B. Isoprenaline
C. Permanent pacemaker
D. Temporary pacemaker
E. No treatment required

Question 10

A 35-year-old previously fit and well man presents with a 2-day history of sharp central chest pain which is worse when lying on his back and is relieved on leaning forwards. Cardiovascular examination, including BP, is normal. His chest X-ray reveals normal lung fields and heart size. His 12-lead

ECG is shown below. The troponin level is measured on admission and is found to be elevated.

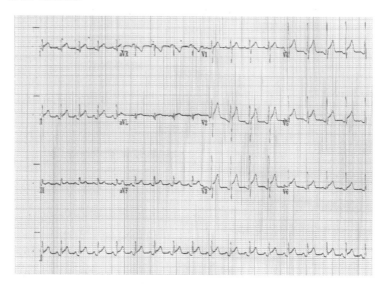

What is your diagnosis?

A. Acute coronary syndrome
B. Pericarditis
C. Myopericarditis
D. Aortic dissection
E. Aortitis

Question 11

A 45-year-old asymptomatic man undergoes routine 12-lead ECG at his GP surgery. The GP feels that his ECG is abnormal and makes a referral to the cardiology outpatient clinic. On examination at the clinic, the man is normotensive with a regular heart rate of 70 beats/min. Cardiovascular examination reveals very quiet heart sounds, although he has a thin chest wall. He undergoes 12-lead ECG, which is taken by the clinic nurse.

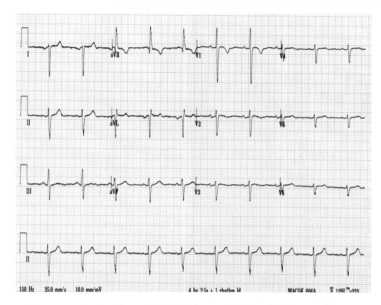

However, after looking at the ECG the cardiologist decides to take another recording himself. This second ECG is shown below:

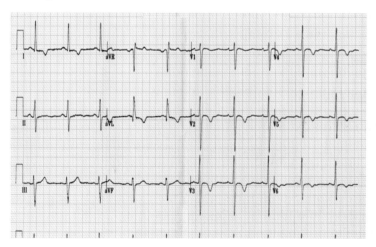

What is the diagnosis?
A. Pericardial effusion
B. Pericarditis
C. Dextrocardia
D. First-degree heart block
E. WPW syndrome

Question 12

A 19-year-old asymptomatic athlete undergoes a routine cardiovascular evaluation organised by his club to exclude any underlying cardiac conditions. He is normotensive with no family history of sudden death. The cardiovascular examination reveals normal heart sounds. His 12-lead ECG is shown below:

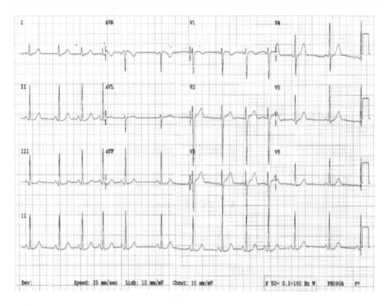

What striking change is seen on the ECG?
A. First-degree heart block
B. WPW syndrome
C. Long QTc interval
D. Sinus arrhythmia
E. Wandering pacemaker

Question 13

A 58-year-old man is seen by his GP with symptoms of palpitations. He has a history of myocardial infarction and hypertension. He is on aspirin, ramipril, simvastatin and glyceryl trinitrate (GTN) spray. Cardiovascular examination reveals normal heart sounds. His 12-lead ECG performed at the GP surgery while having palpitations is shown below:

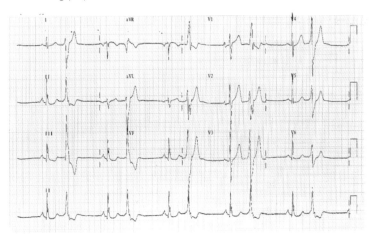

What is the diagnosis?
A. Sinus arrhythmia
B. Atrial bigeminy
C. Ventricular bigeminy
D. Supraventricular ectopic beats
E. Ventricular ectopic beats

Question 14

A 45-year-old man is admitted to the CCU following successful thrombolysis of an inferior myocardial infarction. He has been stable and asymptomatic with a BP of 120/80 mmHg. However, the CCU nurses notice a sudden drop in his heart rate with a peculiar ECG pattern. They perform a 12-lead ECG, the results of which are shown:

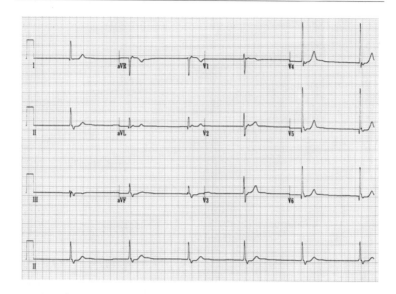

1. What is the diagnosis based on the ECG findings?
A. Complete heart block
B. Second-degree heart block
C. Junctional rhythm
D. Sinus bradycardia
E. First-degree heart block

2. What will be your management strategy?
A. IV amiodarone
B. Close observation
C. Temporary pacemaker insertion
D. Permanent pacemaker insertion
E. Isoprenaline infusion

Question 15

A 40-year-old Afro-Caribbean male has been complaining of headache and recurrent epistaxis for the past 3 months. He has also noticed that his breathing is getting laboured, especially on exertion. He has a strong family history of stroke. He has been a lifelong non-smoker and does not consume alcohol. On examination, he has normal heart sounds but his BP is elevated to

160/95 mmHg. He thinks high BP is probably from the anxiety of seeing doctors. His 12-lead ECG performed at the clinic is shown below:

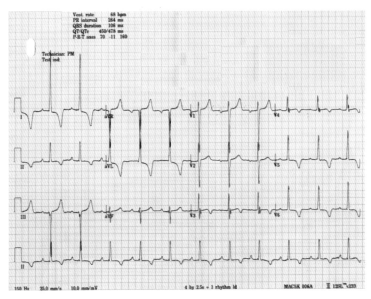

Based on his ECG, what structural abnormalities are likely to be present on the echocardiogram (choose two from the following)?
A. Left atrial enlargement
B. Left ventricular hypertrophy
C. Left ventricular dysfunction
D. Right ventricular hypertrophy
E. Ventricular septal defect
F. Atrial septal defect
G. Pericardial effusion

Question 16

A 65-year-old man who was recently diagnosed with heart failure secondary to dilated cardiomyopathy was prescribed bisoprolol and candesartan. He was still in NHYA class 2–3 symptoms of heart failure. Subsequently his community heart failure nurse starts him on an aldosterone antagonist (spironolactone). There is a remarkable improvement in his symptoms and exercise tolerance.

Two weeks later, he undergoes a routine ECG at the GP surgery, which is shown below:

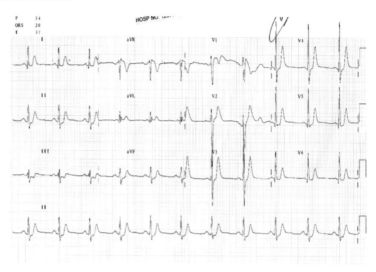

Based on his ECG, what blood test should his GP request?

A. Full blood count

B. Renal function test

C. Liver function test

D. Thyroid function test

E. Bone profile

Question 17

A 64-year-old woman presents to her GP surgery with a 2-hour history of central chest discomfort and shortness of breath. At the GP surgery she looks unwell, and is sweating, cold and clammy. Her GP performs an immediate ECG (shown) and subsequently calls the ambulance to send her to A&E.

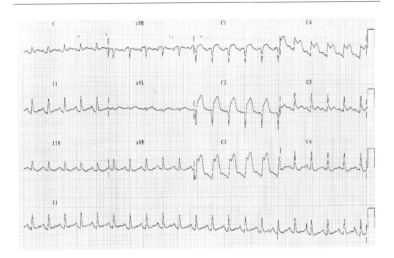

What is the diagnosis based on the ECG finding?

A. Anterior ischaemia

B. Inferoposterior myocardial infarction

C. Inferior myocardial infarction

D. Posterior myocardial infarction

E. Anterior myocardial

Question 18

A 21-year-old man who plays for a local football club is referred to the cardiology outpatient clinic with two episodes of syncope while playing football. On questioning, he complains of several episodes of palpitations and dizzy spells over the past 2 months. He had not revealed his symptoms previously because he was worried he would not be selected for a forthcoming football tournament. His father had died suddenly at the age of 30 years while refereeing a football match. The cause of his father's death following the post-mortem examination was reported as 'myocardial infarction.'

Cardiovascular examination reveals harsh ejection systolic murmur in the left sternal edge with normal blood pressure. Prior to his arrival, he underwent a 24-hour ambulatory ECG recording organised by his GP, which exhibited several runs of non-sustained ventricular tachycardia that corresponded with his symptoms of palpitations. His 12-lead ECG is shown:

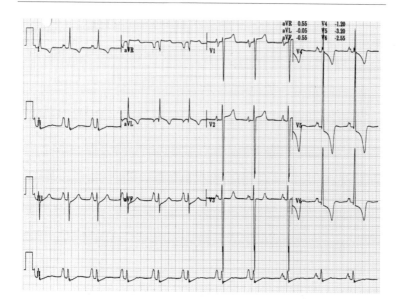

What is your working diagnosis based on his presentation and ECG?

A. Aortic stenosis

B. Hypertrophic cardiomyopathy

C. Dilated cardiomyopathy

D. Restrictive cardiomyopathy

E. Infective endocarditis

Question 19

An 85-year-old man presents to A&E with symptoms of dizzy spells and two episodes of documented syncope. He is not on any regular medications and has no significant past medical history. On examination, he is normotensive with heart rate of 40 beats/min. He has normal heart sounds on cardiovascular examination. His 12-lead ECG performed in the clinic is shown:

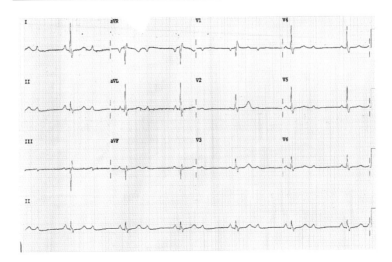

What is the diagnosis based on his ECG and presentation?

A. Complete AV block
B. Mobitz type 1 AV block
C. Mobitz type 2 AV block
D. First-degree heart block
E. Bifascicular block

Question 20

A 45-year-old smoker with a history of hypertension presents to A&E with a 12-hour history of central crushing chest pain. On arrival at A&E, he is pain-free, but looks extremely unwell. His heart rate is 95 beats/min with a systolic BP of 80 mmHg. Cardiac auscultation reveals normal heart sounds, but he has bi-basal inspiratory crackles in the chest. The 12-lead ECG performed at admission is shown:

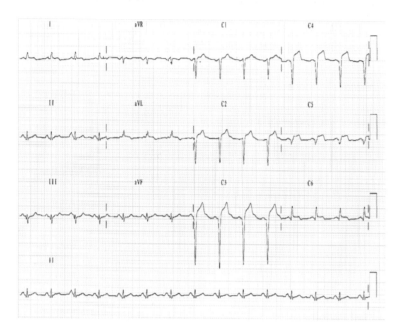

He had arthroscopy for his left knees 4 months earlier and an ECG performed prior to this procedure is found in his old notes and is shown below:

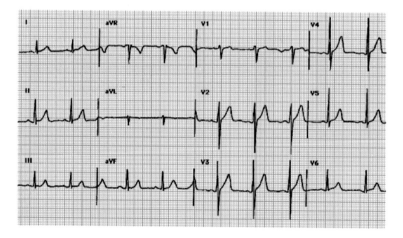

1. Comparing his previous and current ECGs, what is the probable diagnosis?

A. Acute ST-elevation myocardial infarction
B. Completed anterior myocardial infarction
C. Inferior myocardial infarction
D. There are no major changes noted
E. Inappropriate lead positioning on his chest wall

2. Why is he currently unwell?

A. Septic shock
B. Cardiogenic shock
C. Pericardial effusion
D. Myocarditis
E. Dehydration

Question 21

A 65-year-old woman who has been previously treated for breast carcinoma presents with progressively worsening shortness of breath. She has no previous cardiac history. On examination, she is tachycardic with heart rate of 120 beats/ min and a BP of 120/70 mmHg. She has elevated jugular venous pressure, but her lung bases are clear. Her chest X-ray is shown below:

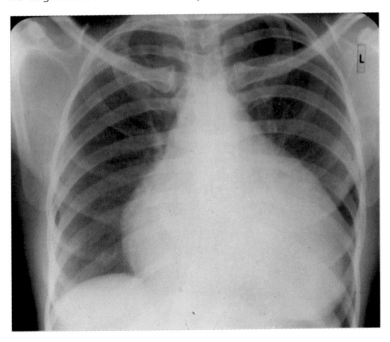

What is the diagnosis?

A. Pericardial effusion
B. Cardiac tamponade
C. Myocarditis
D. Constrictive pericarditis
E. Restrictive cardiomyopathy

Cardiac Medicine

Answers

Question 1

1. B *Inferior myocardial infarction*

The ECG shows ST-segment elevation in inferior precordial leads (II, III and aVF) suggestive of an acute ST-elevation myocardial infarction (STEMI) involving the inferior wall of left ventricle (LV).

It is important to know leads that represent various walls of ventricle on the 12-lead ECG:

- The precordial leads V1–V4 represent the anterior and septal walls of the left ventricle.
- Leads II, III and aVF represent the inferior wall.
- Leads I, aVL and V5–V6 represent the lateral wall.
- V1-V2 represents a mirror reflection of the posterior wall.
- Right-sided leads ($V1^R$ –$V6^R$) represent the right ventricular wall.

2. B *Primary angioplasty*

There are two forms of treatment for acute ST-elevation myocardial infarction. The traditional treatment has been IV thrombolysis. However, primary angioplasty has been now accepted as the better treatment option. It involves an angiogram and subsequent treatment of the culprit lesion with the use of stents. There have been many trials showing the superiority of primary angioplasty over the traditional use of thrombolytic agents. Most hospitals in the UK provide primary angioplasty service, though some hospitals still use thrombolysis due to lack of facilities and manpower.

Question 2

1. E *Complete AV block*

The ECG shows that there is no relationship between the P waves and QRS complexes. Atria and ventricles are beating at their own pace. On the ECG, P-waves can be seen marching over QRS complex, ST-segment and sometimes on T-waves (as shown by the arrows), producing distorted complexes, very classical of complete AV block

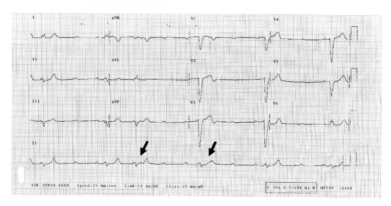

2. C *Permanent pacemaker*

Complete AV block is treated with the insertion of a permanent pacemaker (PPM) without which patients are at a risk of asystole and sudden death. PPM is inserted via the cephalic or subclavian vein under local anaesthesia.

If the patient with complete heart block has haemodynamic compromise in the form of low BP, dizzy spells or acute confusion, then a temporary pacemaker is inserted until the permanent system is implanted. A temporary pacemaker can be a potential source of infection which can be fatal. It should be inserted only if there are signs of haemodynamic compromise. Moreover, temporary pacemaker carries a risk of cardiac perforation especially in the hands of inexperienced operators.

Atropine and isoprenaline can be used as an alternative to a temporary pacemaker; however, they may not be successful in all patients. These drugs can be used in situations when there are no operators for a temporary pacemaker or in the presence of inexperienced operators.

Question 3

1. B *Anterolateral myocardial infarction*
The ECG exhibits ST-segment elevation in all the precordial and lateral limb leads suggestive of extensive anterolateral myocardial infarction. Reciprocal changes are quite classical of ST-elevation myocardial infarction and in this case are seen in the inferior leads (as ST-segment depression).

2. C *Acute pulmonary oedema*
The chest X-ray shows the classic bat-wing appearance suggestive of accumulation of fluid in the interstitial lung spaces. This is likely to be due to poor left ventricular function resulting from massive anterolateral myocardial infarction. The mainstay of treatment is to offload fluid from the lungs with the use of IV furosemide and a GTN infusion. Once stable from heart failure, the patient should be started on beta-blockers and angiotensin-converting enzyme (ACE) inhibitors or angiotensin receptor blockade to improve symptoms and prevent mortality.

Question 4

1. B and E *Right bundle branch block and sinus tachycardia*
The ECG shows presence of RSR' pattern (tall R wave) in lead V1 with prolonged QRS complex (>120 ms), suggestive of right bundle branch block. There are clear P waves before every QRS complexes (shown by arrows) and the heart rate is >100 beats per minute to suggest sinus tachycardia.

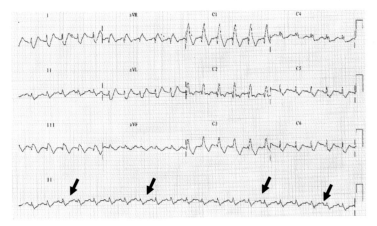

2. C *Acute pulmonary embolism (PE)*

This is a classical presentation of acute PE. There is evidence of severe hypoxia with a relatively normal looking chest X-ray, which cannot account for the degree of hypoxia. The presence of sinus tachycardia with right bundle branch block on the ECG points towards acute strain on the right heart.

The patient should undergo an urgent CT-pulmonary angiogram to diagnose the condition. If the diagnosis confirms PE, patient should be treated with thrombolysis in view of his haemodynamic compromise.

Question 5

1. C *Ventricular tachycardia (VT)*

The ECG shows broad complex regular tachycardia. The possible differential diagnosis includes VT or supra-ventricular tachycardia with aberrancy. In the background of recent myocardial infarction or LV dysfunction, all broad complex tachycardias should be treated as VT.

2. D *Emergency direct current cardioversion (DCCV)*

In view of haemodynamic compromise, VT should be treated with an emergency DCCV. In the absence of haemodynamic compromise, VT could be treated pharmacologically (amiodarone, beta-blocker).

Question 6

1. B *Atrial fibrillation (AF)*

The 12-lead ECG shows narrow complex tachycardia, which is irregularly irregular, diagnostic of AF. Systemic hypertension, ischaemic heart disease and valvular heart disease (especially mitral valve diseases) are the commonest pathological conditions that can predispose to AF.

2. B *Beta-blocker*

According to the published NICE guidelines (2005), the first drug of choice in controlling ventricular rate in AF is the beta-blocker. The second choice is the calcium channel blockers, and digoxin is preferred in sedentary individuals (usually in elderly patients) or patients who are intolerant to beta-blockers and calcium channel blockers. The commonly used beta-blockers are bisoprolol and metoprolol due to their cardio-selective properties.

3. C *Warfarin*

The lady in question is at a higher risk of thromboembolic phenomenon from AF. The commonly used score to decide the need for warfarin is the CHADS2 score.

C – congestive heart failure (1)
H – hypertension (1)
A – age ≥ 75 years (1)
D – diabetes mellitus (1)
S2 – stroke or transient ischaemic attack (TIA) (2)

Each of these factors is given a certain score (as shown in the brackets). Patients with AF with CHADS2 score >1 qualify for warfarin. If they score 1 or <1 they can be treated with aspirin or clopidogrel. However, prescription of warfarin has to be the decision of the treating clinician, as elderly patients with a risk of recurrent falls may not be appropriate candidates for warfarin, even if they have a high CHADS2 score.

Question 7

1. A *Supraventricular tachycardia*
The 12-lead ECG shows regular narrow complex tachycardia.

Any tachycardia with a narrow complex is termed supraventricular tachycardia (implying their origin is above the ventricle). If the narrow complex tachycardia is regular, the differential diagnosis includes atrial flutter with 2:1 block or AV-nodal re-entry tachycardias. The AV-nodal tachycardia could be one of the following:
- Intra-AV nodal re-entry tachycardia
- Extra-AV nodal re-entry tachycardia.

Intra-AV nodal tachycardia is due to presence of dual pathway within the AV-node. Extra-AV nodal re-entry tachycardia is commonly due to the presence of accessory pathway (an extra electrical connection between atria and the ventricle).

Irregular narrow complex tachycardia is usually due to atrial fibrillation.

One way to differentiate between atrial flutter and AV nodal re-entry tachycardias is to transiently block the AV node using drugs such as IV adenosine/beta-blocker or calcium-channel blocker.If the tachycardia is due to atrial flutter, saw-toothed flutter waves can be witnessed following AV-node blockage. In contrast, a flat line is observed on blocking the AV-node in AV-nodal re-entry tachycardia and it usually terminates the arrhythmia by breaking the circuit.

2. A WPW type ECG

The second ECG after cardioversion shows a short PR interval and delta waves suggestive of pre-excitation. The cause of pre-excitation is due to accessory pathway between the atria and the ventricle. It can potentially form a circuit between the atria and ventricle, which are then susceptible for the generation of supraventricular tachycardia, as was the case in this patient.

3. C Radiofrequency ablation

Accessory pathway leading to SVT warrants permanent ablation of the pathway using radiofrequency technology, which is usually performed by an electrophysiologist.

Question 8

D Intracardiac defibrillator

The ECG exhibits prolonged QTc-interval (>500 ms). The upper limit for QTc interval in females is 460 ms. Given her symptoms, family history of sudden death and prolonged QTc interval on ECG, she probably has congenital long QT syndrome (Jervell and Lange–Nielsen syndrome variant). Congenital long QT syndromes (LQTS) are the group of inherited cardiac conditions that result from the mutations involving various ion channels of the cardiac myocytes, predominantly the potassium and sodium channels.

Two clinical phenotypes have been described in LQTS that vary with the type of inheritance and the presence or absence of sensorineural hearing loss:
1. The autosomal dominant form, the Romano–Ward syndrome, has a pure cardiac phenotype.
2. The autosomal recessive form, the Jervell and Lange–Nielsen syndrome, which is associated with LQTS and sensorineural deafness, has a more malignant clinical course.

Congenital LQTS are one of the well-known causes of sudden cardiac death. Individuals with LQTS are prone to develop polymorphic VT and subsequently sudden death. Any symptomatic patients with a background of family history of sudden death warrant intracardiac defibrillator.

There is no role for electrophysiological studies in LQTS.

Question 9

1. C Tri-fascicular block

This woman's ECG shows three prominent features: right bundle branch block, first-degree AV block and left axis deviation. Combination of these features is termed as a trifascicular block. Presence of trifascicular block indicates a faulty conduction system at various levels, such as the AV node and His-bundles. It can lead to pauses and cause symptoms of dizzy spells and syncope.

2. C Permanent pacemaker[1]
Symptoms of dizzy spells and/or syncope in the presence of trifascicular block warrants permanent pacemaker placement.

Question 10

C Myopericaditis
History is vital in the diagnosis of pericarditis and this patient reports classic symptoms of pericarditis. The patient's ECG shows a global ST elevation, which is one of the classical changes seen in pericarditis. Moreover, the patient has elevated myocardial enzymes, suggesting that the inflammatory process has involved the myocardium in addition to the pericardium and hence is termed myopericarditis. The patient should undergo echocardiogram to assess left ventricular function, which can be impaired. Another reason to request an echocardiogram is to look for pericardial effusion, which is a commonly associated with pericarditis / myopericarditis. A small percentage of individuals with myopericarditis can develop dilated cardiomyopathy, which is a more serious condition. Thus patients require monitoring with follow up echocardiograms a few weeks or months after the initial episode to assess the left ventricle.

Question 11

C Dextrocardia
The first ECG shows indeterminate axis or extreme axis deviation. When there is malposition of limb leads whilst performing the ECG, it can lead to indeterminate axis, which is termed technical dextrocardia. However, in technical dextrocardia there is appropriate progression of the R waves across the chest leads (V1-V6). In this case, the progression of the R wave is poor as evidenced by decreasing amplitude of R wave across the chest leads. This indicates that the patient has true dextrocardia. The cardiologist might have suspected this and has performed an ECG by placing the leads on the right side; the subsequent ECG shows appropriate progression of the R wave across the chest leads.

Question 12

D Sinus arrhythmia

The ECG shows variation between the R–R intervals in the background of a sinus rhythm. The changing interval is as a result of respiratory variation. This is a classic description of sinus arrhythmia, which is quite commonly seen in athletes and young people. This is an example of a physiological arrhythmia and does not need any further investigations or treatment. The arrhythmia disappears on subjecting the individual to a brief period of exercise.

Question 13

C Ventricular bigeminy

The ECG shows regular ectopic complexes after every sinus beat, which is termed bigeminy. Since the QRS complexes of the ectopic beats are prolonged (>120 ms), it is originating from the ventricle and hence termed ventricular bigeminy.

Bigeminy can occur in patients with or without structural heart disease. The commonest cause of bigeminy is ischaemic heart disease and/or LV dysfunction. The drugs that are used to abort symptomatic bigeminy are beta-blockers. If patients are not symptomatic, no treatment is necessary, especially with a structurally normal heart.

Question 14

1. C Junctional rhythm

The ECG shows bradycardia and if you observe the QRS complexes closely, there are P waves buried within the QRS complexes. This suggests that the impulses are being generated in the AV node, and reach both atrium and ventricles simultaneously. Since the atrium is being depolarised from below (at the AV node), the P waves are negative in the inferior leads.

2. B Close observation

Junctional rhythm can be encountered in patients following inferior myocardial infarction. The right coronary artery usually supplies the SA node, and occlusion of the artery can cause ischaemia or infraction of node leading to its dysfunction. The AV node can take over the function by generating the impulse, but at a lower rate than the normal sinus rate. On most occasions, nodal rhythm can be a transient phenomenon, as the SA node can recover from ischaemia. If patients are haemodynamically stable, observation alone can be sufficient. However, if patients fail to recover from nodal rhythm, insertion of a permanent pacemaker should be considered.

Question 15

A Left ventricular hypertrophy (LVH); B left atrial enlargement
This patient has voltage criteria for LVH (S-wave in V1 + R-wave in V5 or V6 < 35 mm on the ECG). An isolated voltage criterion is not a sensitive marker for LVH. However, presence of other signs such as left axis deviation, ST-segment depression in the lateral leads and left atrial enlargement makes LVH more likely. The left atrial enlargement causes prolongation of the terminal part of P wave, which causes P-waves to appear as a 'M' in the inferior leads and as a more negative P wave in lead V1 (as seen in the ECG). The appearances of the notched P wave in lead II is also termed as 'P mitrale'. The P wave should be >0.12 ms (three small squares) in the inferior leads and the negative component in lead V1 should be >0.1 mV (one small square) to indicate left atrial enlargement. A negative P-wave in V1 is a more sensitive indicator of left atrial enlargement than P mitrale.

Question 16

B Renal function test
The ECG shows tall-tented T waves, suggestive of hyperkalaemia. The cause of hyperkalaemia in this case is due to the combination of an ACE inhibitor and an aldosterone antagonist. If the potassium is found to be elevated on a blood test, the triggering medications should be stopped and patient should be treated with intra-venous insulin and dextrose to reduce serum potassium levels.

Question 17

C Anterior myocardial infarction
The ECG shows ST elevation in the anterior leads (V1-V4), which is suggestive of anterior myocardial infarction. The best intervention for ST-elevation myocardial infarction is primary angioplasty (see question 1).

Question 18

B Hypertrophic cardiomyopathy (HCM)
The ECG shows tall QRS complexes with ST depression and deep T-wave inversions in the lateral leads. These features are quite classical of the presence of LVH (as per the Romilt–Estes criteria). With a family history of sudden death,

the boy's recurrent episodes of syncope and auscultation of ejection systolic murmur point firmly towards the diagnosis of hypertrophic cardiomyopathy (HCM).

Hypertrophic cardiomyopathy is a primary myocardial disorder characterised by the presence of LVH in the absence of a local or systemic cause, such as aortic stenosis or hypertension. It is due to the mutations involving various parts of contractile proteins of cardiac myocytes. HCM is one of the commonest causes of sudden cardiac death in young individuals (<40 years).

Question 19

C Mobitz type 2 AV block
The ECG shows that every second P wave is not followed by a QRS, which suggests that there is a 2:1 block in the AV node. Identification of a Mobitz type 2 AV block, with symptoms is an indication for insertion of a permanent pacemaker. Haemodynamically compromised patients require insertion of temporary pacemaker prior to permanent pacing system.

Question 20 *20a: 2, 20b: 2*

1. B Completed anterior myocardial infarction
The ECG shows pathological Q wave in the anterior leads (V1–V4) suggestive of a previous myocardial infarction. Given his history, it probably suggests that the patient suffered an anterior myocardial infarction when he experienced chest pain of 12 hours' duration. The ECG from 4 months previous, shows R waves across the anterior chest leads, suggesting the most likely cause of his current ECG changes is a completed anterior myocardial infarction.

2. Cardiogenic shock
The patient is hypotensive after a massive anterior myocardial infarction, which makes it more likely that his cardiac output is significantly compromised. The presence of cardiogenic shock in the background of myocardial infarction is an ominous sign and needs immediate attention. Administration of IV fluids for hypotension can actually make his situation worse and should be given with caution.

Question 21

A Pericardial effusion

The chest X-ray shows a large globular heart, which in conjunction with an elevated jugular venous pressure and her clinical presentation, raises the suspicion of pericardial effusion. The diagnosis has to be confirmed with an echocardiogram. Given the history of breast carcinoma, the likely cause for the effusion is malignancy.

Clinically there is no evidence of haemodynamic compromise, which favours the diagnosis of pericardial effusion over that of cardiac tamponade. Patients with cardiac tamponade are extremely unwell and have additional features of hypotension and pulsus paradoxus (a drop of at least 10 mmHg in arterial blood pressure on inspiration).

2 Respiratory Medicine

Questions

Saleem I.M. Khoyratty and Santino Jacob Capocci

Question 1

Consider the following graph depicting lung volumes and answer the questions below.

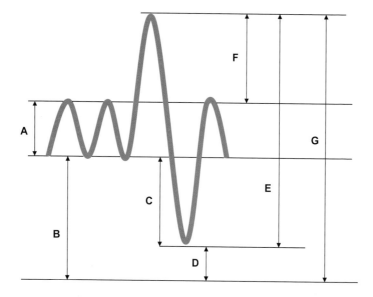

Clinical Data Interpretation for Medical Finals: Single Best Answer Questions, First Edition.
Edited by Philip Socrates Pastides and Parveen Jayia.
© 2012 Philip Socrates Pastides and Parveen Jayia. Published 2012 by John Wiley & Sons, Ltd.

1. Which dimension on the graph represents functional residual capacity?

A. A
B. B
C. C
D. D
E. E
F. F
G. G

2. Which dimension on the graph represents inspiratory reserve volume?

A. A
B. B
C. C
D. D
E. E
F. F
G. G

3. Which dimension on the graph represents tidal volume?

A. A
B. B
C. C
D. D
E. E
F. F
G. G

4. Which dimension on the graph represents residual volume?

A. A
B. B
C. C
D. D
E. E
F. F
G. G

5. Which dimension on the graph represents expiratory reserve volume?

A. A
B. B
C. C
D. D
E. E
F. F
G. G

6. Which dimension on the graph represents total lung capacity?

A. A
B. B
C. C
D. D
E. E
F. F
G. G

7. Which dimension on the graph represents vital capacity?

A. A
B. B
C. C
D. D
E. E
F. F
G. G

Question 2

1. What is the approximate tidal volume of a 70 kg male?

A. 100 mL
B. 450 mL
C. 700 mL
D. 2400 mL
E. 5000 mL

2. What is the approximate total lung capacity of a 70 kg male?

A. 2 L
B. 4 L
C. 6 L
D. 7 L
E. 10 L

3. What is the approximate vital capacity of a 70 kg male?
A. 1 L
B. 3 L
C. 4.5 L
D. 7 L
E. 10 L

4. What is the approximate volume of the anatomical dead space in a 70 kg male?
A. 50 mL
B. 100 mL
C. 150 mL
D. 200 mL
E. 250 mL

Question 3

1. Which of the following would cause a rightward shift in the oxygen dissociation curve?
A. A drop in temperature
B. An increase in carbon monoxide
C. A decrease in carbon dioxide
D. A drop in pH
E. A decrease in 2,3-diphosphoglycerate (2,3-DPG)

2. Which of the following would cause a leftward shift in the oxygen dissociation curve?
A. Increased 2,3-DPG
B. An increase in temperature
C. An increase in carbon monoxide
D. An increase in carbon dioxide
E. A drop in pH

Question 4

A 72-year-old man presents to A&E saying he has been feeling generally unwell over the past few weeks. You are the on-call FY2. After examining the patient you request a chest X-ray, which is shown:

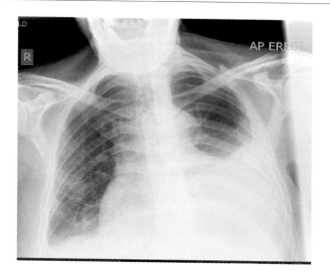

1. Which of the following features would you not expect to find on examination?

A. Stony dullness on percussion on the left side
B. Tracheal deviation towards the left side
C. Dyspnoea
D. Decreased tactile vocal fremitus on the left side
E. Decreased breath sounds on the left side

The patient is admitted to have the pleural effusion drained. The results of the pleural tap are as follows:
pH – 7.16
Glucose – 0.4
LDH – 11 200 IU/L
Protein – 46 g/L (serum protein 64)

2. What is the next most appropriate step?

A. Await pleural cytology
B. Send pleural rheumatoid factor
C. Prescribe antibiotics and refer for pleural drainage in the next few days
D. Start tuberculosis treatment
E. Prescribe antibiotics and refer for pleural drainage immediately

Question 5

A 73-year-old man presents to A&E short of breath for the past 3 days. He complains of a productive cough of yellow/green sputum. He is on regular inhalers and is a lifelong smoker with a 100 pack/year history. He has gained no relief from his inhalers and so called the ambulance.

He arrives at A&E on 15 L/min of oxygen. You note that his respiratory rate is 28/min and his saturations are 100%. He has good chest expansion and has bilateral breath sounds with a widespread expiratory wheeze throughout both lung fields. You receive the following arterial blood gas (ABG):

Inspired oxygen concentration – 15 L/min rebreathe bag
pH – 7.22
PO_2 – 43.03 kPa
PCO_2 – 9.27 kPa
HCO_3 – 24.7 mEq/L
Base excess – +0.7 mmol/L
Lactate – 1.5 mmol/L
You compare this to his previous discharge ABG on 21% oxygen:
pH – 7.37
PO_2 – 11.6 kPa
PCO_2 – 5.5 kPa
HCO_3 – 22.5 mEq/L
Base excess – −1.5 mmol/L
Lactate – 0.7 mmol/L

1. What is the cause of the patient's acidosis?
A. Respiratory
B. Metabolic
C. Mixture of respiratory and metabolic
D. Sepsis
E. None of the above

2. What would you do next?
A. Stop supplementary oxygen, use room air for 20 min and repeat the ABG
B. Use controlled oxygen with saturations of between 88 and 92% for 20 min and repeat the ABG
C. Give nebulisers, steroids and controlled oxygen with saturations between 88 and 92% and repeat the ABG in 1 hour
D. Start non-invasive ventilation
E. Intubate the patient

You start the patient on controlled oxygen therapy to maintain saturations of 88–92% (28%) and repeat the ABG after 60 min. The results of the ABG are as follows:

Inspired oxygen concentration – 28%
pH – 7.3
PO_2 – 8.4 kPa
PCO_2 – 8.2 kPa
HCO_3 – 25.4 mEq/L
Base excess – +3.4 mmol/L
Lactate – 1.4 mmol/L

3. What is the best management of this patient's ventilation?
A. Sign a DNAR (do not attempt resuscitation) form
B. Non-invasive ventilation
C. Intubation
D. Use 24% controlled oxygen
E. Use 40% controlled oxygen

Question 6

A 28-year-old asthmatic patient comes to A&E. He states that he has been increasingly short of breath for the last 5 days, and has been trying to cope on his salbutamol, beclomethasone and salmeterol inhalers, with little benefit. He states that he was particularly short of breath overnight and hence called an ambulance this morning.

On examination you note that the patient has a respiratory rate of 20, on auscultation you hear very little air entry bilaterally and surprisingly only a minimal wheeze is audible. You take an ABG on room air and receive the following result:

pH – 7.37
PCO_2 – 5.9 kPa
PO_2 – 6.9 kPa
HCO_3 – 25.4 mEq/L
Base excess – +0.9 mmol/L
Lactate – 1.8 mmol/L
Sats – 90%

What do you do next?

A. The patient has no wheeze, so send the patient home with advice to return if he deteriorates

B. Give the patient back-to-back nebulisers, steroids and call the medical registrar and discuss with ITU immediately

C. Give the patient a salbutamol nebuliser and reassess

D. Give the patient some antibiotics

E. Send the patient for a chest X-ray to rule out a pneumothorax

Question 7

You see a 68-year-old in A&E who complains of sudden-onset pleuritic chest pain which started the previous day, 3 weeks after her total knee replacement operation. She complains of swelling of her leg on the operation side for the past 4 days. There is no contraindication to anticoagulation.

The patient looks short of breath, blood pressure is normal and you find little else on examination. An ECG shows the following:

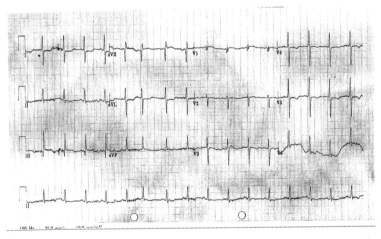

A chest X-ray shows no abnormalities. You perform an ABG and get the following result on room air:

Inspired oxygen concentration – 21%

pH – 7.5

PCO_2 – 2.6 kPa

PO_2 – 8.9 kPa

HCO_2 – 19.5 mEq/L

Base excess – −4.0 mmol/L

Sats – 91%

What is the next most appropriate step to manage this patient?
A. D-dimer, and await the result
B. Start oxygen, start low-molecular-weight heparin and refer to the medical registrar as a potential pulmonary embolism
C. Thrombolyse
D. Start controlled oxygen and see if she improves
E. Observe

Question 8

A 47-year-woman lady attends her GP surgery having felt gradually more unwell over the last 3 months. She complains of increasing shortness of breath, although she is still able to complete all her usual activities of daily living. This has worsened to the extent where, the previous night and this morning, she had two episodes of haemoptysis on each occasion.

She also complains of recurrent sinus problems and previously came to see you 4 years ago requesting a referral to an ENT specialist for rhinoplasty.

Investigations show the following:
Urine dipstick – blood ++ and protein +
Hb – 10.3 g/dL
WCC – 6.8×10^9/L
Platelets – 376×10^9/L
Na – 140 mmol/L
K – 4.9 mmol/L
Urea – 16.8 mmol/L
Creatinine – 278 mmol/L

What additional blood test would you request?
A. TFT (thyroid function tests)
B. Serum bHCG
C. Interferon gamma release assay
D. ANCA
E. HIV antibody

Question 9

A 45-year-old man who has sex with men attends A&E complaining of increased shortness of breath. He has been suffering from this for the past 6 weeks and it is mainly affecting him when he is doing daily activities.

On examination his pulse is 67 and regular with a blood pressure of 110/65 mmHg. You note oral thrush. Respiratory rate is 18 at rest, but this increases to 28 on minimal exertion. Saturations are 97% on room air, decreasing to 87% on walking. Respiratory examination is otherwise unremarkable.

A chest radiograph shows bilateral pulmonary infiltrates.

What is the most likely diagnosis?

A. Pneumocystis pneumonia
B. Community-acquired pneumonia
C. Recurrent pulmonary embolism
D. Pneumothorax
E. Pleural effusion

Question 10

A 25-year-old woman, who has recently arrived from India, attends her G.P.'s surgery complaining of increasing lethargy over the past two months. Upon further questioning she gives a good history of increased shortness of breath and night sweats causing her to change her pyjamas during the night. She also complains of a cough, productive of yellow sputum.

She is currently living in a hostel in East London until she can gather enough money to rent somewhere else, but denies knowing anybody with similar symptoms. Her two children are currently asymptomatic.

On examination the patient is currently apyrexial, has a pulse rate of 98 beats per minute (regular) and a blood pressure of 98/49 mmHg. Her saturations (on room air) are 95% and her respiratory rate is 17 breaths per minute.

Auscultation of the chest reveals harsh breath sounds in the right upper zone.

1. What is the most definitive, appropriate next investigation?

A. Chest X-ray
B. Sputum sample
C. Full blood count
D. Spirometry
E. Echocardiogram

2. What would be the most appropriate treatment?

A. Quadruple therapy with anti-tuberculous medication for 1 week

B. Quadruple therapy with anti-tuberculous medication for 1 year

C. Moxifloxacin for 1 week

D. Clarithromycin and amoxicillin for 1 week

E. Quadruple therapy with anti-tuberculous medication for 2 months, with dual therapy for another 4 months

Question 11

A 75-year-old patient attends her rheumatology outpatient clinic. She suffers from severe rheumatoid arthritis and has failed treatment with many standard rheumatoid medications (prednisolone, methotrexate, sulphasalazine). She is still complaining of severe joint pain which is inhibiting an otherwise normal lifestyle.

Her rheumatologist decides to start her on infliximab and invites her to re-attend the clinic in 3 months. Upon re-attending she is much happier with the state of her rheumatoid arthritis and says that her joint problems have almost disappeared. She is still complaining of fatigue and malaise, however, and states that while this improved at first, it has now become her primary problem. She also complains of a nagging cough that is productive of sputum.

What is the most likely diagnosis?

A. Upper respiratory tract infection

B. *Streptococcus pneumoniae* pneumonia

C. *Staphylococcus aureus* pneumonia

D. *Mycobacterium tuberculosis* infection

E. Adverse reaction to infliximab

Question 12

A 46-year-old Afro-Caribbean woman attends her GP surgery complaining of a 4-month period of increasing dyspnoea, weight loss, fatigue and a dry cough. Over the last week she has developed some non-specific joint pains.

She denies any night sweats or rigors, and all other household occupants are well. She denies any history of tuberculosis or any contact with anybody with tuberculosis. She suffers from no other medical conditions and is on no regular medications.

On examination the patient is apyrexial and has normal observations. Auscultation of her chest reveals no abnormalities. The GP does, however, note raised erythematous lesions bilaterally on the anterior part of the lower leg. The GP requests a chest X-ray which shows bilateral hilar shadowing. Blood results are as follows:
Sodium – 143 mmol/L
Potassium – 4.8 mmol/L
Urea – 4.5 mmol/L
Creatinine – 87 mmol/L
Calcium – 2.7 mmol/L
Phosphate – 1.1 mmol/L
Lung function testing:
Forced expiratory volume in 1 s (FEV_1)/forced vital capacity (FVC) – 84%

1. What marker is classically raised with this disease process?
A. C3
B. C8
C. Basophils
D. Angiotensin-converting enzyme
E. Blood glucose

2. What is the likely diagnosis?
A. Tuberculosis
B. Sarcoidosis
C. *S. pneumoniae* infection
D. Legionella pneumonia infection
E. Myeloma

3. What is the treatment?
A. Anti-tuberculous medication for 6 months
B. Anti-tuberculous medication for 12 months
C. Steroids
D. Co-amoxiclav for 1 week
E. Linezolid and vancomycin for 1 week

Question 13

A 76-year-old retired bank manager attends his GP practice complaining of 6 months of increasing breathlessness. He is becoming increasingly worried about this, as only 3 years ago he was running the London marathon. He smoked much earlier in life.

He reports that the breathlessness has gradually increased to the state where he struggles to walk more than 100 m without having to stop. He complains of no other symptoms and has no other medical problems and is on no regular medication. All other family members are well.

On examination the patient has a respiratory rate of 18 and saturations on room air of 92%. He is cyanosed and clubbed. Ausculation of the chest reveals bilateral fine inspiratory crackles.

Lung function test:
FEV_1/FVC – 90%
DLCO – 40% predicted
Arterial blood gas:
pH – 7.44
PO_2 – 7.3 kPa
PCO_2 – 4.0 kPa

What is the likely diagnosis?
A. Mesothelioma
B. Small-cell lung cancer
C. Rheumatoid arthritis-associated lung fibrosis
D. Cystic fibrosis
E. Idiopathic pulmonary fibrosis

Question 14

A 39-year-old male is brought into A&E having been found on the floor by his landlord. He is very confused. The landlord knows the patient relatively well and has been aware of his high alcohol intake, although the patient has been trying to cut back. The patient also suffers from epilepsy that is poorly controlled due to poor compliance with his medications.

On examination the patient has a Glasgow Coma Score(GCS) of 9, he is apyrexial, his respiratory rate is 24 and his other observations are within the normal range. He smells strongly of alcohol and urine. Auscultation of his precordium reveals normal heart sounds, with harsh breath sounds on the right side of the chest.

His blood results are as follows:

Hb – 13.9 g/dL	Sodium – 139 mmol/L
WCC – 15.9 × 10^9/L	Potassium – 4.8 mmol/L
Platelets – 128 × 10^9/L	Urea – 8.9 mmol/L
Neutrophils – 10.8 × 10^9/L	Creatinine – 100 mmol/L

A chest radiograph reveals right-sided opacification with air bronchograms present, obscuring the right heart border.

1. What is the likely diagnosis?

A. Aspiration pneumonia
B. Pleural effusion
C. Hospital-acquired pneumonia
D. Primary lung cancer
E. Lung abscess

2. Which lobe of the lung has been affected?

A. Left upper lobe
B. Left lower lobe
C. Right upper lobe
D. Right middle lobe
E. Right lower lobe

3. What is the treatment for this patient?

A. Observe and when GCS 15 discharge
B. IV co-amoxiclav
C. IV benzylpenicillin and clarithromycin
D. Oral amoxicillin
E. Oral clarithromycin

Question 15

A 73-year-old man attends A&E with an episode of haemoptysis. He reports a couple of smaller episodes over the last couple of days, and says that he was going to see his GP about it. This morning he reports producing about four to five spoonfuls of bright red blood. He says he started to feel increasingly tired over the last couple of months, with increased shortness of breath and a cough. He admits to being a lifelong smoker, smoking about 20 cigarettes per day at the moment, but says he used to smoke up to 60 cigarettes per day respectively during the war.

He suffers from chronic obstructive pulmonary disease(COPD), diagnosed by his GP, and this is generally well controlled on his inhalers. He has never been seen in chest clinic.

On examination he is warm and well perfused, although he looks underweight. You note that he is not clubbed, and auscultation of his chest does not reveal any abnormalities. Investigations are as follows:

Hb – 12.2 g/dL   Sodium – 129 mmol/L
White cell count – 6.9 × 10^9/L   Potassium – 5.0 mmol/L
Platelets – 369 × 10^9/L   Urea – 7.9 mmol/L
Calcium – 2.1 mmol/L   Creatinine – 112 mmol/L

A chest radiograph which reveals a widened mediastinum. This is not seen on a chest radiograph from an admission 8 months ago.

What is the likely diagnosis?

A. Adenocarcinoma of the lung
B. Metastatic secondaries
C. Small-cell lung cancer
D. Aortic dissection
E. foreign body

Respiratory Medicine

Answers

Question 1

1. B

The functional residual capacity is the amount of gas in the lung after normal expiration. It comprises the expiratory reserve volume and the residual volume. Please note that a capacity is formed by the addition of two or more volumes.

2. F

Inspiratory reserve volume is the additional air that can be inhaled after a normal tidal breath in.

3. A

Tidal volume is the amount of air breathed in and out during normal respiration.

4. D

Residual volume is the amount of air left in the lungs after a maximal exhalation.

5. C

Expiratory reserve volume is the amount of additional air that can be breathed out after the end expiratory level of a normal tidal breath.

6. G

Total lung capacity is the volume of gas contained in the lung at the end of maximal inspiration.

7. E

Vital capacity is the amount of air that can be forced out of the lungs after a maximal inspiration.

Question 2

1. B *450 mL*
Tidal volume is approximately 6 mL/kg. Therefore in a 70 kg male this is likely to be around 420 mL, making B the closest and most suitable answer.

2. C *6 L*
Total lung capacity is approximately 80 mL/kg. Therefore in a 70 kg male this should be 5600 mL, making C the closest answer.

3. C *4.5 L*
Vital capacity is approximately 60–70 mL/kg. Therefore in a 70 kg male this is between 4300 and 4900 mL, making C is the closest answer.

4. C *150 mL*
Anatomical dead space is the volume of gas in the conducting airways which is not involved in gas exchange. It is approximately 150 mL.

Question 3

1. D *A drop in pH*
Causes of a right shift include an increase in temperature, an increase in 2,3-DPG, an increase in carbon dioxide a fall in carbon monoxide and a fall in pH (i.e. an increase in H^+ ions). Adult haemoglobin also causes a rightward shift in the oxygen dissociation curve. The mnemonic **CADET** (**c**arbon dioxide, **a**cidosis, 2,3-**D**PG, **e**xercise and **t**emperature) can be used to remember the causes of a rightward shift in the oxygen dissociation curve.

2. C *Increase in carbon monoxide*
Carbon monoxide binds to haemoglobin with 240 times the affinity of oxygen. Haemoglobin can bind four oxygen molecules. Binding of a carbon monoxide molecule at one of these sites, increases the affinity of the oxygen binding at the other sites. This makes it harder for oxygen to dissociate, and therefore a lower partial pressure of oxygen is required for oxygen to be delivered to tissues compared with normal. This is represented as a leftward shift.

Other causes of a leftward shift include reduced temperature, reduced 2,3-DPG, reduced carbon dioxide concentration, alkalosis and the presence of fetal haemoglobin.

Question 4

1. B Tracheal deviation towards the left side

This patient has a left-sided pleural effusion. Apart from answer B, all the other findings are consistent with a left-sided pleural effusion. We can see that the trachea in this case is central. However, if there was any deviation, it would be away from the side with the effusion, as the pressure effect would be greatest on that side.

There are a number of different types of fluid that can accumulate within the pleura. These include fluid, blood (haemothorax), pus (empyema) and chyle (chylothorax).

Broadly, effusions can be split into transudates (caused by a change in starling forces) and exudates (caused by local changes to the production or reabsorption of pleural fluid, e.g. around a pneumonia).

A pleural fluid protein >30 g/L usually distinguishes an exudate from a transudate, but Light's criteria is commonly used to differentiate them if the protein content is borderline. A pleural effusion is defined as an exudate if one of the following is present:

- ratio of pleural protein to serum protein >0.5
- ratio of pleural LDH to serum LDH >0.6
- pleural fluid greater than two-thirds of the normal upper limit for serum LDH (or approximately pleural fluid LDH >200).

It should be remembered that Light's criteria is not 100% accurate (over-diagnoses exudates) and that ultimately assessing the patient and working out the underlying cause will correctly predict the nature of the pleural effusion and is the most accurate method.

Transudates are commonly caused by the 'failures' which will alter Starling's forces to produce a pleural effusion. These would include heart failure (left ventricular failure), liver cirrhosis (hepatic hydrothorax) and fluid overload in renal failure. Transudates also occur with a low serum albumin, nephrotic syndrome, from peritoneal dialysis fluid and in urinothorax (uni-lateral ureteric obstruction). They can occur with hypothyroidism (can be an exudate).

Exudates are commonly caused by malignancy, pulmonary embolism, systemic inflammatory diseases such as rheumatoid arthritis and pneumonia.

The patient does not need to be breathless; however, from looking at the chest X-ray one would expect the patient to be short of breath.

Treatment depends on the underlying cause.

2. E Prescribe antibiotics and refer for pleural drainage immediately
The patient is likely to have an empyema and needs to have this drained as soon as possible. pH < 7.2 (and a low glucose) is consistent with an empyema or infected parapneumonic effusion. The natural history of this means that with time the fluid will loculate and thicken, making it harder to drain. Drainage as soon as possible is indicated. Effusions due to rheumatoid pleurisy can also have a low glucose, as can malignant effusions.

(BTS guideline on investigation of a unilateral pleural effusion in adults – *Thorax* 2010; **65**(Suppl 2): ii4–ii17.)

Question 5

1. A Respiratory
When you compare the ABG on his admission with his previous discharge (baseline) ABG you find that he is now acidaemic. The pCO_2 is raised and the bicarbonate is only now starting to increase to compensate (although it is still within the normal range). His lactate is not raised, so therefore the answer is that his respiratory decline is causing a respiratory acidosis.

A metabolic acidosis would show a low bicarbonate concentration. It could also be due to raised lactate concentration within the blood. A raised lactate is commonly associated with sepsis.

A combination of both respiratory and metabolic causes would lead to a raised carbon dioxide and a low bicarbonate.

2. C Give nebulisers, steroids and controlled oxygen with saturations between 88 and 92% and repeat the ABG in 1 hour
Maintaining saturations between 88 and 92% is sufficient for many COPD patients. The patient has an expiratory wheeze throughout both lung fields, and therefore should be given some nebulisers and steroids. He should be monitored, but, if stable, should have his ABG repeated in 1 hour.

He should be given controlled oxygen and medical treatment for an exacerbation of COPD (nebulisers, steroids and antibiotics if indicated) for 1 hour before considering non-invasive ventilation if he remains acidaemic.

Saturations of 88–92% will allow the patient to remain on the plateau portion of the oxygen dissociation curve. Using air (21% oxygen) may cause the patient to become too hypoxic.

Not giving a patient nebulisers will cause the airways to remain constricted, reducing your ability to oxygenate the patient and remove carbon dioxide.

Intubating the patient would not be your first option, although a discussion with the patient about whether he would like invasive ventilation if he requires it would be a sensible step. Some patients may not want invasive ventilation, and having the discussion with them early can save you having to make the decision for them when they are too unwell.

3. B

The patient has received controlled oxygen to maintain saturations between 88 and 92%. He has received this for 1 hour, which would allow him sufficient time to change his arterial pCO_2. However, his arterial blood gas still shows an acidosis with a raised pCO_2. Provided his chest X-ray does not show a pneumonia (when intubation could be considered) or a pneumothorax (absolute contraindication) and the patient is adequately compliant, he would be suitable candidate for non-invasive ventilation.

A discussion with the patient about resuscitation status again may be sensible, but would not be your next step in the management of the patient's condition.

Intubation would require discussion with the patient and ITU department within your hospital. They would want to know that the patient has been managed optimally on the ward before they would consider bringing the patient up to ITU.

Lowering the patient's oxygen would probably cause the patient to become hypoxic.

Increasing the patient's oxygen concentration will probably cause the patient to become more hypercapnic and therefore more acidotic.

Question 6

B *Give the patient back-to-back nebulisers, steroids and call the medical registrar and discuss with ITU immediately*
The patient has asthma and has a type 1 respiratory failure (low PO_2 with normal pCO_2). The patient should technically have a low pCO_2 as he should be trying to hyperventilate to compensate for his hypoxia. However, after the duration of his exacerbation he is becoming tired, and is not hyperventilating as expected.

You should be immediately worried and call the medical team and ITU to let them know about the patient as he may be a candidate for respiratory support until he overcomes his exacerbation.

Sending the patient home with a hypoxic ABG would be poor practice. The patient, at the very minimum, requires this to be corrected with supplementary oxygen.

Giving the patient a salbutamol nebuliser would be helpful as it would cause bronchodilatation and allow improved oxygenation and removal of carbon dioxide.

Antibiotics may be a good option is the patient has clinical evidence of an infection. However, just giving the patient oxygen without any other treatment would not be the best option.

Clinical examination of the chest has not revealed any signs consistent with a pneumothorax. An X-ray is certainly clinically indicated in this patient (oxygen saturations <92%), but there are other more immediate issues to treat.

Question 7

B *Start oxygen, start low-molecular-weight heparin and refer to the medical registrar as a potential pulmonary embolism*
This patient has a good history for a pulmonary embolism (PE). She has a major risk factor that would cause her to be immobilised. She also complains of symptoms suggestive of a deep vein thrombosis (DVT). She has a tachycardia on her ECG (there may even be S1Q3T3) and there are no chest X-ray signs to suggest a pneumothorax or other cause of her hypoxia.

Her Well's score is 9, which makes her high risk (signs/symptoms of DVT, +3; PE most likely diagnosis, +3; HR >100, +1.5; surgery in the last 4 weeks, +1.5) so a D-dimer is not indicated as it is used to rule out PE in low- and sometimes intermediate-risk patients (depending on the D-dimer assay).

The patient is not unwell enough to be a candidate for first-line thrombolysis (which may be indicated if she were hypotensive and had not recently had an operation). Starting oxygen will help to negate any dead space (ventilated but not perfused lung) caused by the PE, but it will not treat the underlying cause.

Just observing a patient with low saturations and signs of hyperventilation would be bad practice. This patient therefore needs to be referred and requires further investigations for a PE.

If a PE is found, the patient should continue on low-molecular-weight heparin until warfarin has been started and her International Normalised Ratio (INR) or her prothrombin time (PT) is in the therapeutic range. Warfarin inhibits the formation of vitamin K-dependent clotting factors (factors 2, 7, 9 and 10 as well protein C and S) via the inhibition of the production of vitamin K. It does not inhibit any current clotting factors which are already present and this is why is takes a couple of days before the patient will be within the therapeutic range.

Treatment should be continued for 3–6 months.

Question 8

D *ANCA*

This patient has a disease process affecting both her respiratory and her renal systems. Classic diseases that involve these systems together in an examination situation are Wegener's granulomatosis and Goodpasture's syndrome. In this case it is more likely to be Wegener's.

Wegener's is a necrotising granulomatous disease process which can affect the renal and respiratory systems. Within the respiratory system it can cause pulmonary haemorrhage, and within the renal system it can lead to a nephritic process.

Wegener's can affect other systems but classically it affects the sinuses and can lead to nasal deformities. Investigations which can help with the diagnosis of Wegener's include a c-ANCA which is positive. Treatment is with pulsed methylprednisolone and cyclophosphamide.

Goodpasture's syndrome is a disease process caused by antibodies to the glomerular basement membrane. The disease process again affects the respiratory and renal systems and can lead to a similar process to Wegener's. Antibodies to the glomerular basement membrane are positive, while c-ANCA is negative. Treatment is again with immunosuppresion, and in severe cases plasmapheresis may be required.

The other tests are not clinically relevant. Hypothyroidism may cause lethargy and anaemia, but should not cause haemoptysis. An interferon gamma release assay (IGRA) is used to screen for latent tuberculosis infection, not active disease. HIV testing should be considered in any general medical patient. These findings are not consistent with a classic acute seroconversion illness.

Question 9

A *Pneumocystis pneumonia*

This patient most likely has pneumocystis pneumonia (PCP), caused by *Pneumocystis jirovecii* (previously called *Pneumocystis carinii*).

This is a common exam question and a patient at risk of HIV infection or other immunocompromise [including those on transplant immunosuppression, with severe combined immunodeficiency (SCID) or with acute lymphocytic leukaemia] who comes in with dyspnoea and desaturates on exertion warrants a chest X-ray.

Further investigations for this gentleman would include a HIV test and a bronchoscopy or induced sputum. Treatment would include co-trimoxazole, IV pentamidine or clindamycin/primaquine if the patient is allergic to co-trimoxazole. Steroids should be used if the $PaO_2 < 9.3$.

A community-acquired pneumonia would be in your differential diagnosis, but with the classical chest X-ray appearance, high-risk behaviours and classic exertional desaturation, the patient is more likely to have PCP.

The patient is not at high risk for PEs, has chest X-ray changes (you may see a wedge infarct with a massive PE, but otherwise the chest X-ray is normal in these patients) and desaturates on exertion rather than being persistently hypoxic.

The clinical examination and the chest X-ray are not consistent with a pleural effusion or a pneumothorax.

Question 10

1. B *Sputum sample*
2. E *Quadruple therapy with anti-tuberculous medication for 2 months, with dual therapy for another 4 months*

This patient gives a good history for primary pulmonary tuberculosis (TB).

Recent immigrants to the UK have an increased incidence of TB which is about 40 times that of the native population. Spirometry should not be performed in patients who are at high risk of having smear-positive TB for infection control reasons.

It is not uncommon for patients to present in an asymptomatic fashion, although this patient has many of the classic signs and symptoms and has the additional risk factor of living in a hostel.

TB is caused by *Mycobacterium tuberculosis*. It classically affects the lungs (about 75%) in the primary infection and can cause signs and symptoms such as:

• Malaise
• Weight loss
• Fever
• Night sweats
• Cough
• Haemoptysis.

Diagnosis is made by culturing the organism classically from sputum samples which are stained with Ziehl–Neelsen or auramine to reveal acid-fast bacilli.

The organism may be cultured on a Lowenstein–Jensen culture medium, but this is a very slow process. Polymerase chain reaction (PCR) is a newer, faster method of diagnosing the disease.

A full blood count may give you some information about the inflammatory response, but would not give you any more diagnostic information. An echocardiogram does not give you any more diagnostic information.

A chest X-ray is definitely indicated, and may show that an infective process is ongoing within the right apex, but will not give a clear diagnosis in this case.

Treatment depends on the area of the body affected by the organism. For pulmonary TB a 6-month course of anti-tuberculous medication is recommended. This comprises of the mnemonic **RIPE**:

- **R**ifampicin
- **I**soniazid
- **P**yrazinamide
- **E**thambutol.

Depending on sensitivities and clinical improvement, pyrazinamide and ethambutol are usually discontinued after 2 months, with rifampicin and isoniazid being continued for a total of 6 months. [Note: standard abbreviations for TB medications are R (rifampicin), H (isoniazid), Z (pyrazinamide), E (ethambutol)].

Multi-drug-resistant TB is becoming an increasing issue and is defined as TB resistant to both rifampicin and isoniazid. HIV antibodies should be tested routinely.

Answers A and B have the wrong treatment regimes. Moxifloxacin for 1 week would start to treat TB, but as a single agent would predispose to drug resistance (and hence would be contraindicated).

Clarithromycin and amoxicillin are used in the treatment of bacterial community-acquired pneumonia.

Question 11

D Mycobacterium tuberculosis infection
This is an exam favourite: a patient being started on infliximab (a monoclonal antibody against tumour necrosis factor) which causes an improvement with the primary disease state but leads to reactivation of TB.

A chest X-ray should have been performed before initiating treatment and another chest X-ray can now be performed and compared. If positive, the patient should have sputum cultures sent off, but should be started on anti-tuberculous treatment.

An upper respiratory tract infection is a possibility. However, the patient is producing sputum and, with the other clinical history and in an exam, this would not be the main thing to rule out.

Options B and C would again be a possible differential diagnosis, but with the clinical history TB is the greatest concern.

There is no sign of an allergic reaction. The patient has no outward signs of an allergic reaction and has been taking the medication for 3 months.

Question 12

1. D *Angiotensin-converting enzyme*
2. B *Sarcoidosis*
3. C *Steroids*

This patient has sarcoidosis. Sarcoidosis is a multi-system non-caseating granulomatous disease. The disease has no known cause.

Classically patients present in exam questions with malaise, fatigue, a *dry* cough and erythema nodosum (the skin lesion found on the shins of this patient). A number of other systems may be involved leading to arthralgia, anterior uveitis, parotid enlargement, keratoconjunctivitis and diabetes insipidus.

Investigations classically will show a raised serum calcium. This is caused by an increased production of 1,25-dihyroxycholecalciferol (1,25-DHCC) which leads to an increased plasma calcium concentration. Serum angiotensin-converting enzyme (ACE) may also be raised and a chest X-ray will typically reveal bilateral hilar lymphadenopathy.

Candidates should be aware of Lofgren's syndrome which comprises bilateral hilar lymphadenopathy, erythema nodosum and arthralgia.

Management of sarcoidosis is initially with steroids if hypercalcaemia, cardiac, eye and joint problems, bothersome respiratory symptoms or progressive respiratory impairment are present. The disease may warrant steroid-sparing agents such as methotrexate.

Question 13

E *Idiopathic pulmonary fibrosis*

Idiopathic pulmonary fibrosis (IPF, previously also known as cryptogenic fibrosing alveolitis, CFA) is an idiopathic lung condition which presents with dyspnoea, clubbing and fine bilateral inspiratory crackles.

The patient is an ex-smoker of many years, making lung cancer unlikely in an exam setting. The history gives no occupational exposure to asbestos and no other conditions suggestive of rheumatoid arthritis. The patient also does not complain of cough.

Investigations have shown a restrictive lung pattern and a type 1 respiratory failure, both consistent with IPF.

Further investigations to confirm the diagnosis would include a high-resolution CT scan (HRCT). This scan takes thin slices at fixed intervals and allows much finer images to be obtained of the lung parenchyma that can miss small focal lesions such as small lung tumours. An open lung biopsy is sometimes used if the diagnosis is not completely clear on the CT.

Treatment is usually supportive. Oxygen is used if hypoxic, although some clinicians advocate a trial of a combination of azathioprine, low-dose steroids and N-acetylcysteine to see if this slows the deterioration in lung function.

Question 14

1. A *Aspiration pneumonia*
2. D *Right middle lobe*
3. B *IV co-amoxiclav*

This patient has a pneumonia, likely to be secondary to aspiration. The patient has a couple of risk factors for aspirating, including his alcohol use and his epilepsy that is poorly controlled.

The patient has a consolidative process confirmed on the chest X-ray. With the additional risk factors (history of drinking and epilepsy), covering for an aspiration would be sensible, and therefore anaerobic cover would be warranted.

Co-amoxiclav consists of amoxicillin and clavulanic acid. The two components work together, with the clavulanic acid acting as an alternative substrate for the beta-lactamase, which would otherwise confer resistance to the amoxicillin.

Co-amoxiclav offers anaerobic cover as well as good Gram-positive cover. IV benzylpenicillin and clarithromycin offer no anaerobic cover.

The chest X-ray shows a consolidative process (air bronchograms) obscuring the right heart border, the classic sign for a right middle lobe process.

Question 15

C *Small-cell lung cancer*

The extensive history of smoking as well as weight loss, fatigue and haemoptysis all suggest a malignant process. The investigations reveal a rapidly progressing lung lesion, the low sodium could be due to syndrome of inappropriate antidiuretic hormone hypersecretion (SIADH) or hypoadrenalism (Addison's) due to metastases.

With the patient's extensive smoking history, and the rapid progression of the lesion on chest radiograph, a small-cell lung cancer is the likely diagnosis.

All lung cancers are associated with smoking, but adenocarcinoma is the most common lung cancer among patients who have never smoked. Clubbing is less common with small-cell lung cancers. Hypercalcaemia is associated with squamous cell cancers due to the secretion of parathyroid hormone-related peptide (PTHrP).

Management will depend on a combination of factors, including the stage of the cancer, the performance status of the patient and, of course, the patient's wishes. For small-cell lung cancer the prognosis is poor, especially without chemotherapy.

With the prominent smoking history a lung primary malignancy is most likely. With an aortic dissection, the patient would probably be very unwell. There is no suggestion of ingestion of a foreign body.

3 Haematology

Questions

Philip S. Pastides, Parveen Jayia and Neil Chauhan

Question 1

Consider the blood film below:

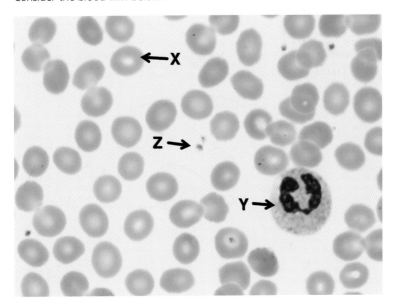

1. What is cell X?

A. Erythroblast
B. Erythrocyte
C. Reticulocyte
D. Sickle cell
E. Pencil cell

Clinical Data Interpretation for Medical Finals: Single Best Answer Questions, First Edition.
Edited by Philip Socrates Pastides and Parveen Jayia.
© 2012 Philip Socrates Pastides and Parveen Jayia. Published 2012 by John Wiley & Sons, Ltd.

2. What is cell Y?

A. Neutrophil
B. Lymphocyte
C. Eosinophil
D. Monocyte
E. Basophil

3. What is structure Z?

A. Red cell fragment
B. Malarial parasite
C. Platelets
D. Spherocyte
E. Howell–Jolly body

Question 2

The red cells in the following film are abnormal:

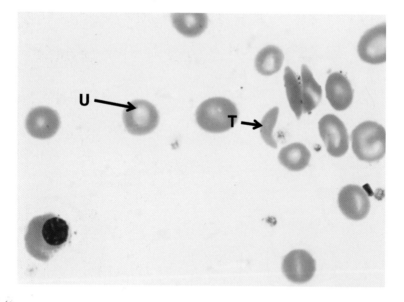

1. What is cell T?

A. Pencil cell
B. Target cell
C. Sickle cell
D. Spherocyte
E. Elliptocyte

2. What is structure U?

A. Red cell fragment
B. Malarial parasite
C. Platelet
D. Spherocyte
E. Howell–Jolly body

Question 3

Consider the film below:

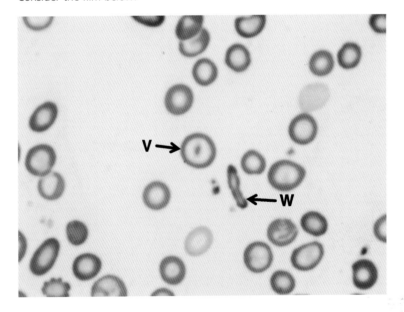

1. What is cell V?

A. Pencil cell
B. Target cell
C. Sickle cell
D. Spherocyte
E. Elliptocyte

3. What is cell W?

A. Pencil cell
B. Target cell
C. Sickle cell
D. Spherocyte
E. Elliptocyte

Question 4

A 32-year-old woman visits her GP due to ongoing nausea and tiredness. She is pleasantly surprised to discover that she is pregnant. On examination she looks a bit pale, so the GP performs some blood tests to investigate further. These are shown below:

		Range
White cell count (WCC)	5.0×10^9/L	$3.8–11.8 \times 10^9$
Haemoglobin (Hb)	8.1 g/dL	11.5–16.5
Platelets	274×10^9/L	$150–400 \times 10^9$
Haematocrit	0.249 L/L	0.37–0.50
Mean cell volume (MCV)	106 fL	78–100
Neutrophils	2.75×10^9/L	$2.00–6.77 \times 10^9$
Lymphocytes	2×10^9/L	$1–4 \times 10^9$
Monocytes	0.5×10^9/L	$0.2–0.8 \times 10^9$
Eosinophils	0.04×10^9/L	$0.04–0.40 \times 10^9$
Basophils	0.01×10^9/L	$0.01–0.10 \times 10^9$

What is the most likely haematological cause for her anaemia?

A. Iron deficiency
B. Folate deficiency
C. Chronic disease
D. Sideroblastic anaemia
E. Thalassaemia trait

Question 5

A 41-year-old housewife visits her GP complaining of 2 months of fatigue and shortness of breath on exertion. Her periods have been irregular for the last year and heavier than normal. On examination she appears pale and has pale mucous membranes. Her full blood count is shown below:

		Range
White cell count	6.9×10^9/L	$3.8–11.8 \times 10^9$
Haemoglobin (Hb)	6.3 g/dL	11.5–16.5
Platelets	640×10^9/L	$150–400 \times 10^9$
Haematocrit	0.222 L/L	0.37–0.50
Mean cell volume	62 fL	78–100
Neutrophils	3.8×10^9/L	$2.00–6.77 \times 10^9$
Lymphocytes	2.7×10^9/L	$1–4 \times 10^9$
Monocytes	0.28×10^9/L	$0.2–0.8 \times 10^9$
Eosinophils	0.07×10^9/L	$0.04–0.40 \times 10^9$
Basophils	0.07×10^9/L	$0.01–0.10 \times 10^9$

Analysis of her blood film reveals anisocytosis, microcytosis and hypochromia. Target cells are occasionally seen throughout the film.

What is the most likely haematological diagnosis?
A. Folate deficiency anaemia
B. B12 deficiency anaemia
C. Iron deficiency anaemia
D. Thalassaemia
E. Sideroblastic anaemia

Question 6

A 63-year-old woman presents to her GP complaining of fatigue. On examination she looks very pale. Her cardiovascular system is unremarkable but she is noted to have decreased sensation in both legs below the knee and absent ankle jerks. An urgent full blood count shows the following (range in brackets):

Hb – 8.6 g/dL (13.0–16.5)
MCV – 136 fL (80–100)
WCC – 3.8×10^9/L ($4–11 \times 10^9$)
Platelets – 116×10^9/L ($150–400 \times 10^9$)

What is most likely haematological diagnosis?
A. Iron deficiency anaemia
B. Folate deficiency
C. Vitamin B12 deficiency
D. Thyrotoxicosis
E. Bone marrow failure

Question 7

A 56-year-old man complains of long-standing symptoms of tiredness and shortness of breath on exertion. He has a 30-year history of hypertension for which he has been on thiazide and calcium channel blocker medications for the last 15 years. On examination he looks pale. His blood pressure is 165/111 mmHg. His apex beat appears displaced laterally. His lung fields appear clear and there are no signs of pedal or sacral oedema. Retinal screening revealed a grade III retinopathy. His latest investigations results are shown below:

White cell count (WCC)	5.0×10^9/L	$3.8–11.8 \times 10^9$
Haemoglobin (Hb)	8.7 g/dL	11.5–16.5
Platelets	201×10^9/L	$150–400 \times 10^9$
Haematocrit	0.264 L/L	0.37–0.50
MCV	86 fL	78–100
Neutrophils	2.75×10^9/L	$2.00–6.77 \times 10^9$
Lymphocytes	2×10^9/L	$1–4 \times 10^9$
Monocytes	0.5×10^9/L	$0.2–0.8 \times 10^9$
Eosinophils	0.04×10^9/L	$0.04–0.40 \times 10^9$
Basophils	0.01×10^9/L	$0.01–0.10 \times 10^9$
Sodium	139 mmol/L	135–145
Potassium	5.4 mmol/L	3.5–5.1
Urea	36.7 mmol/L	3–8
Creatinine	465 mmol/L	60–125

Blood film – anisocytotic normochromic cells
Bone marrow aspirate – normal cellularity. No specific diagnostic features. Normal iron stores
Chest X-ray – cardiomegaly
ECG – sinus rhythm, left ventricular hypertrophy

What is the most likely haematological cause of his anaemia?

A. Iron deficiency
B. B12 deficiency
C. Chronic disease
D. Folate deficiency
E. Aplastic anaemia

Question 8

Which of the following blood count profiles is consistent with a patient with iron deficiency anaemia?

	1	2	3	4	5
Serum iron (11.5–16.5 g/dL)	10.1	10.1	10.1	10.1	10.1
Total iron-binding capacity (250–370 µg/dL)	450	450	300	200	160
Serum ferritin (20–250 µg/L)	125	5	160	5	280

A. 1
B. 2
C. 3
D. 4
E. 5

Question 9

A 6-month-old Bangladeshi boy is noted to be pale by his GP at a routine visit. His mother had noted an occasional jaundice. On examination he looks pale with pale mucous membranes. He also has a palpable liver and spleen. He is sent for blood tests which are shown below:

White cell count	11.4×10^9/L	$3.8–11.8 \times 10^9$
Haemoglobin (Hb)	6.8 g/dL	11.5–16.5
Platelets	310×10^9/L	$150–400 \times 10^9$
Haematocrit	0.172 L/L	0.37–0.50
MCV	60.4 fL	78–100
Neutrophils	6.27×10^9/L	$2.00–6.77 \times 10^9$
Lymphocytes	4.5×10^9/L	$1–4 \times 10^9$
Monocytes	0.57×10^9/L	$0.2–0.8 \times 10^9$
Eosinophils	0.11×10^9/L	$0.04–0.40 \times 10^9$
Basophils	0.04×10^9/L	$0.01–0.10 \times 10^9$
Ferritin	142 mg/L	40–380
Bilirubin	27 mmol/L	3–17

Examination of his blood film reveals target cells and an increased proportion of reticulocytes. Haemoglobin electrophoresis shows raised A2 and a haemoglobin F level of 85% (normal <1%).

What is the most likely haematological diagnosis?

A. Iron deficiency anaemia
B. Thalassaemia
C. Sickle cell disease
D. Folate deficiency
E. Autoimmune haemolytic anaemia

Question 10

A 19-year-old West African student consumes a large amount of alcohol in a nightclub. In the early hours of the morning he develops severe abdominal pain and is brought to A&E by an ambulance crew. He denies any significant past medical or family history. On examination he is in obvious pain, sweating and anxious. His abdomen is tender with generalised guarding; however, bowel sounds are present. The on-call surgical team reviews the patient with a view to taking him to theatre for a laparotomy. His investigations are shown below:

White cell count	8.9×10^9/L	$3.8–11.8 \times 10^9$
Haemoglobin (Hb)	8.9 g/dL	11.5–16.5
Platelets	437×10^9/L	$150–400 \times 10^9$
Haematocrit	0.267 L/L	0.37–0.50
MCV	87.9 fL	78–100
Neutrophils	5.9×10^9/L	$2.00–6.77 \times 10^9$
Lymphocytes	2.5×10^9/L	$1–4 \times 10^9$
Monocytes	0.36×10^9/L	$0.2–0.8 \times 10^9$
Eosinophils	0.22×10^9/L	$0.04–0.40 \times 10^9$
Basophils	0.09×10^9/L	$0.01–0.10 \times 10^9$

His urea, electrolytes, amylase and coagulation screen are normal. His blood film shows sickle cells, target cells and Howell–Jolly bodies. An arterial blood gas on air was unremarkable.

What is the most likely diagnosis?

A. Surgical abdomen requiring laparotomy
B. Sickle cell crisis
C. Biliary colic
D. Gastritis
E. Pancreatitis

Question 11

A 16-year-old girl visits her GP complaining of a sore throat and a low-grade fever over the last few days. She is up to date with all her vaccines. Her blood film is shown below:

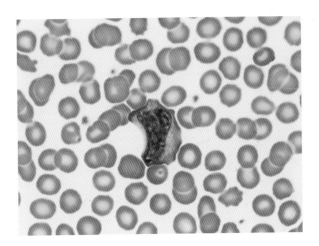

Examination she is found to have enlarged tender cervical lymph nodes and an inflamed pharyngeal mucosa. A full blood count shows:

Hb – 13.2 g/dL (13.0–16.5)
MCV – 96 fL (80–100)
WCC – 13.8 × 10⁹/L (4–11 × 10⁹)
Lymphocytes – 6.2 × 10⁹/L (1–4 × 10⁹)
Platelets – 116 × 10⁹/L (150–400 × 10⁹)

What is the most likely diagnosis?

A. Infectious mononucleosis
B. Leukaemia
C. Influenza
D. Tonsillitis
E. Lymphoma

Question 12

This 56-year old man presented to A&E with sudden onset of numbness and weakness in his right arm and leg, which resolved after 10 minutes. His full blood count is shown below. His ECG revealed normal sinus rhythm.

White cell count	13.6×10^9/L	$3.8–11.8 \times 10^9$
Haemoglobin (Hb)	21.2 g/dL	11.5–16.5
Platelets	478×10^9/L	$150–400 \times 10^9$
Haematocrit	0.72 L/L	0.37–0.50
MCV	83.3 fL	78–100
Neutrophils	10.23×10^9/L	$2.00–6.77 \times 10^9$
Lymphocytes	1.72×10^9/L	$1–4 \times 10^9$
Monocytes	0.60×10^9/L	$0.2–0.8 \times 10^9$
Eosinophils	0.28×10^9/L	$0.04–0.40 \times 10^9$
Basophils	0.15×10^9/L	$0.01–0.10 \times 10^9$

What is the underlying cause of his condition?

A. Lymphoma
B. Polycythaemia rubra vera
C. Acute myeloid leukaemia
D. Bacterial meningitis
E. Agranulocytosis

Question 13

A 1-year-old boy presents to hospital with repetitive and prolonged nose bleeds. Initially they were related to falls but now they have become spontaneous. He has a series of blood tests as follows:

Haemoglobin (Hb)	12.1 g/dL	11.5–16.5
Platelets	490×10^9/L	150–400
Prothrombin time	14 s	12–15 s
Activated partial thromboplastin time (APTT)	114 s	28–38 s
Thrombin Time	12 s	12–15 s
Factor VIIIC	<0.006 IU/mL	28–38 s
von Willebrand Factor (vWF)	1.30 IU/mL	12–15 s
Platelet aggregation	Normal	

What is the most likely haematological diagnosis?
A. Idiopathic thrombocytopenic purpura
B. Haemophilia A
C. Haemophilia B
D. Disseminated intravascular coagulopathy
E. Von Willebrand's disease

Question 14

A 60-year-old lady presents to A&E with left lower limb swelling 10 days after undergoing a hip replacement. She has a past medical history of osteoarthritis and is on paracetamol for pain relief post-surgery but no other medication. The left calf is tender, hot and swollen. Peripheral pulses are present. She is neither tachypnoeic nor dyspnoeic. Her chest is clear, her oxygen saturations are 100% on room air and her blood pressure is 140/80 mmHg. The FY1 asks you what treatment to give while diagnostic tests are organised for the following morning.

What is the most appropriate treatment?
A. No treatment
B. Treatment dose low-molecular-weight heparin
C. Warfarin anticoagulation
D. Prophylactic dose low-molecular-weight heparin
E. Thrombolysis

Question 15

A 23-year-old woman is rushed to hospital after a ruptured ectopic pregnancy. She is taken to theatre immediately and treated successfully surgically. However, due to the large loss of blood, she receives a 10-unit transfusion. She is haemodynamically stable on the ward. A postoperative coagulation screen is performed, the results of which are shown below:

Haemoglobin (Hb)	10.1 g/dL	11.5–16.5
Platelets	68×10^9/L	$150–400 \times 10^9$
Prothrombin time	20 s	12–15 s
APTT	58 s	28–38 s
Thrombin time	21 s	12–15 s
Fibrinogen	1.2 g/L	1.5–4.0

What is the most likely haematological diagnosis?
A. Idiopathic thrombocytopenic purpura
B. Haemophilia A
C. Result of massive blood transfusion
D. Essential thrombocytopenia
E. Bone marrow failure

Question 16

A 34-year-old pedestrian is hit by a car and thrown into the air. He is brought in to A&E in a drowsy state. His blood pressure is 97/67 mmHg and he is tachycardic at 112 beats/min. The left side of his chest is not moving and is dull to percussion. His abdomen is rigid. He is given 2 L of IV fluids and a chest drain is inserted into the left chest, which drains 1 L of blood. Despite these measures, he remains haemodynamically unstable. His full blood count and coagulation screen are shown below:

White cell count	28.7×10^9/L	$3.8–11.8 \times 10^9$
Haemoglobin (Hb)	6.7 g/dL	11.5–16.5
Platelets	21×10^9/L	$150–400 \times 10^9$
Haematocrit	0.214 L/L	0.37–0.50
MCV	93 fL	78–100
Neutrophils	22.6×10^9/L	$2.00–6.77 \times 10^9$
Lymphocytes	5.2×10^9/L	$1–4 \times 10^9$
Monocytes	0.57×10^9/L	$0.2–0.8 \times 10^9$
Eosinophils	0.03×10^9/L	$0.04–0.40 \times 10^9$
Basophils	0.03×10^9/L	$0.01–0.10 \times 10^9$
Prothrombin time	38 s	12–15 s
APTT	98 s	28–38 s
Thrombin time	21 s	12–15 s
D-dimers	9.0 mg/L	<0.25

The blood film shows fragmented red blood cells.

What is the most likely haematological diagnosis?
A. Idiopathic thrombocytopenic purpura
B. Haemophilia A
C. Haemodilution effect
D. Disseminated intravascular coagulopathy
E. Von Willebrand's disease

Question 17

Consider the following X-ray:

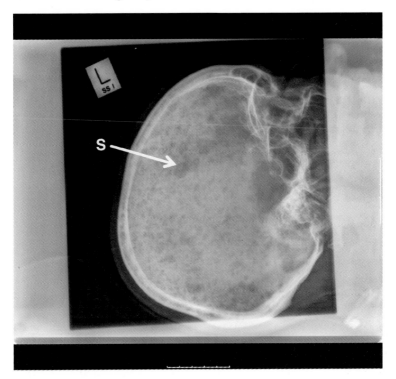

What is the likely pathological process identified by S?

A. Extramedullary haemopoesis
B. Lytic lesion
C. Chloroma
D. Lymphomatous deposit
E. Bony metastases

Question 18

A previously fit and well 70-year-old man presents with confusion to A&E. His daughter mentions a recent history of lower back pain for which he has been taking analgesia. His urine dipstick shows the following:
Blood – negative
Protein – +++

Leucocytes – negative
Nitrites – negative
His blood results are as follows:

Hb – 10.5 g/dL

WCC – 8.2×10^9/L

Platelets – 148×10^9/L

MCV – 100 fL

Neutrophils – 5.7×10^9/L

Urea – 15 mmol/L

Creatinine – 220 mmol/L

Total serum protein – 82 g/L

Albumin – 30 g/L

Calcium – 2.7 mmol/L

   An X-ray confirms an L2 wedge fracture.

What is the most likely diagnosis?

A. Urinary tract infection

B. B12 deficiency

C. Non-specific anti-inflammatory drug-induced renal failure

D. Hodgkin's disease

E. Myeloma

Question 19

An 8-year-old girl presents to her local A&E with a 2-week history of increasing fatigue, shortness of breath on exertion and pallor. On examination her chest is clear, there is no lymphadenopathy, and her spleen is not palpable. Her skin is noted to have multiple flat red sports that do not fade on pressing and fading bruises. She is afebrile with no signs of an infection. Her blood count is as follows:

Hb – 8 g/dL

WCC – 150×10^9/L

Platelets – 24×10^9/L

Neutrophils – 5×10^9/L

C-reactive protein (CRP) – 2 mg/L

Her blood film is shown. A decision is made by your consultant to transfer her to the local Children's hospital.

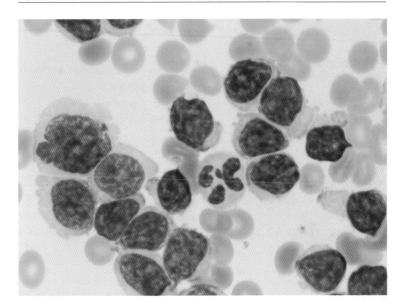

What is the most likely provisional diagnosis?

A. Meningitis
B. Chronic lymphocytic leukaemia (CLL)
C. Acute myeloid leukaemia (AML)
D. Chromic myeloid leukaemia (CML)
E. Acute lymphoblastic leukaemia (ALL)

Question 20

*The following five patients have had a group and save performed. The results
are shown below:*

Patient	Cell surface groups			Serum group cells		
	Anti-A	Anti-B	Anti-D	A cells	B cells	O cells
A	− −	− −	+ +	+ +	+ +	− −
B	+ +	+ +	− −	− −	− −	− −
C	+ +	− −	− −	− −	+ +	− −
D	− −	− −	− −	+ +	+ +	+ +
E	+ +	− −	+ +	− −	+ +	− −

1. **Which patient is blood group A Rh D–?**
2. **Which patient is blood group AB Rh D–?**
3. **Which patient has blood group O Rh D+?**

Haematology

Answers

Question 1

1. B *Erythrocyte*

Erythrocytes, also known as a red cells, contain haemoglobin which give their characteristic colour. They are biconcave discs to maximise oxygen capacity and under a microscope show a pale centre. They are the only cells in the body without a nucleus, losing them as part of their maturation process.

2. A *Neutrophil*

Neutrophils are easily identifiable on normal blood films, being the most common white cell. They have multi-lobed nuclei and contain granules. Their role is to fight infection.

3. C *Platelets*

Platelets appear as small fragments that have an important role in haemostasis.

Question 2

1. C *Sickle cell*

This red cell has taken an unusual shape. It has contracted and looks like a boat or sickle due to it containing haemoglobin S (a haemoglobin variant where a point mutation has replaced glutamine with valine). It is characteristic of sickle cell disease.

2. E *Howell–Jolly body*

The red cells in this film show singular black dots which are called Howell–Jolly bodies. They represent DNA fragments that the spleen would ordinarily remove from mature red cells. They are therefore found in patients who have either undergone splenectomy or who are functionally hyposplenic, such as in sickle cell disease.

Question 3

1. B *Target cell*
This red cell has a 'bull's eye' appearance with the normal central pallor having an extra dot of redness. This happens with red cell disorders, liver dysfunction and some medications.

2. A *Pencil cell*
Note the elongated characteristic shape of a pencil cell. These cells are often seen in association with iron deficiency.

Question 4

B *Folate deficiency*
With a raised MCV, this anaemia is macrocytic in nature. Pregnancy also depletes folate levels and this needs to be replaced, as a decreased folate level in pregnancy can lead to neural tube defects for the developing foetus. For this reason women planning to conceive are recommended to take folate supplements.

Question 5

C *Iron deficiency anaemia*
This lady is suffering from iron deficiency anaemia secondary to menorrhagia. The MCV is low, making it a microcytic anaemia, thereby excluding answers A and B. If she was suffering with sideroblastic anaemia, then the diagnostic feature of ring sideroblasts (marrow red cell precursors) with a ring of iron granules surrounding the nucleus would be present.

Thalassaemia would present earlier and with different clinical features. You may have noted the reactive rise in platelets (reactive thrombocytosis) which further supports the diagnosis.

Her blood film (in Question 3) confirms the anaemia with much fewer red cells than normal (as in Question 1). The red cells are small (microcytic) and there is variation in size and shape (anisocytosis and poikilocytosis). There are pencil shapes and target cells in keeping with the diagnosis.

She needs to be started on iron replacement therapy and investigated for the cause of her menorrhagia.

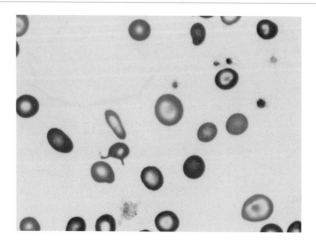

Question 6

C Vitamin B12 deficiency

This patient is clearly anaemic, both clinically and biochemically. Other than fatigue and pallor, clinical signs could include a large, 'beefy' tongue. Since the MCV is raised, this is a macrocytic anaemia and characteristic changes in the blood and bone marrow would show megaloblastic changes, hence the term megaloblastic anaemia. The blood film would show large red cells and hypersegmented neutrophils (see below).

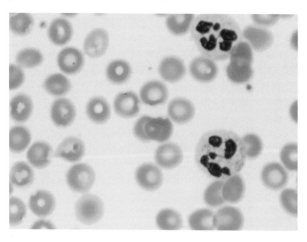

This and the neurological changes would be in keeping with a B12 deficiency.

B12 is absorbed at the terminal ileum. Pernicious anaemia is the most common cause of vitamin B12 deficiency. Other causes include low dietary intake, malabsorption disorders and inflammatory bowel disease, especially Crohn's disease. Vitamin B12 deficiency can cause peripheral neuropathy and, potentially, severe and irreversible damage to the nervous system.

Diagnosis is made by demonstrating low B12 with the presence of low intrinsic factor and autoantibodies to gastric parietal cells. The Schilling test is rarely used now. Treatment involves replacement of B12 with intramuscular injections and treating any identifiable cause.

Question 7

C *Chronic disease*
This patient clearly has long standing renal failure secondary to cardiovascular disease or hypertension with evidence of systemic involvement (cardiomegaly and retinopathy). His MCV is normal this excluded answers A, B and D. He has also had a bone marrow aspirate which was unremarkable, thus making answer E less likely. In this case, this patient will be unlikely to benefit from iron replacement but could be considered for erythropoietin therapy if his blood pressure is controlled.

Question 8

B 2
Iron deficiency can easily be diagnosed by reviewing the blood counts and requesting haematinic studies. In iron deficiency anaemia, the serum iron is low, total iron-binding capacity is high and serum ferritin is low.

Question 9

B *Thalassaemia*
This young child is showing signs of beta-thalassaemia. It is predominantly prevalent around the Mediterranean basin, but due to migration, the majority of new UK cases are of South Asian heritage. He has a microcytic anaemia with a normal ferritin level. His bilirubin is raised and clinically he has hepatosplenomegaly with episodes of jaundice, suggestive of haemolysis. His haemoglobin F, continues to remain high due to the inability to form normal haemoglobin which would ordinarily suppress fetal haemoglobin.

Question 10

B *Sickle cell crisis*

Sickle cell disease is an autosomal dominant genetic blood disorder characterized by red blood cells that can assume an abnormal, rigid, sickle shape which decreases the cells' flexibility.

A 'sickle cell crisis' is used to describe acute conditions occurring in patients with sickle cell disease. Triggers include infection, dehydration, hypoxia, alcohol and anxiety. A vaso-occlusive crisis is caused by sickle-shaped red blood cells that obstruct capillaries and restrict blood flow to an organ, resulting in ischaemia, pain, necrosis and often organ damage

Diagnosis is made on blood film and haemoglobin analysis which show sickle-shaped cells and other features of hyposplenism, such as Howell–Jolly bodies (basophilic nuclear remnants in circulating erythrocytes that tend to be removed by a normal spleen). The haemoglobin electrophoresis will reveal the presence of haemoglobin S (HbS).

The blood film below (as in Question 2) shows sickle and target cells in keeping with a haemoglobinopathy. There are Howell–Jolly bodies and nucleated red bloods cells due to the hyposplenism.

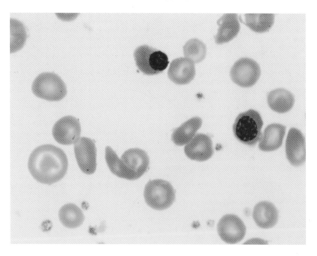

Treatment of the crisis is supportive with fluid rehydration, analgesia and oxygen. In the long term, patients tend to stay on prophylactic antibiotics and folic acid in an attempt to decrease the likelihood of further episodes. They require chronic care management in conjunction with specialist centres given the range of complications they can develop.

Question 11

A Infectious mononucleosis

Infectious mononucleosis, or 'kissing disease', is an infectious viral disease caused by the Epstein–Barr virus (EBV). It is transmitted via the oral route. Symptoms of this condition include a sore throat, fever, fatigue, weight loss, malaise, pharyngeal inflammation, petechiae and anorexia. Common signs include lymphadenopathy and splenomegaly.

It is usually diagnosed clinically but confirmatory tests looking for specific EBV antibodies or a positive heterophil reaction (Monospot test) can be done to confirm the diagnosis.

Blood films show characteristic changes in EBV infection (and other viral infections) such as reactive lymphocytes as shown below. Treatment is supportive as the condition is usually self-limiting.

Question 12

B Polycythaemia rubra vera

This patient has presented with symptoms suggestive of a transient ischaemic attack (TIA). From his full blood count we can see he has a marked rise in haemoglobin, but also in the overall white cell and platelet numbers. This and the neurological history suggest a diagnosis of polycythaemia rubra vera (primary polycythaemia). Confirming signs would include splenomegaly and a characteristic bone marrow examination. The vast majority of polycythaemia rubra vera patients carry the Jak II mutation (95%).

The rise in red cells causes an increase in blood viscosity. Patients are more prone to blood clots and so can present with venous thromboembolism or arterial thrombi causing myocardial infarction or cerebral vascular accidents.

There is no cure for the condition at present and treatment focuses on managing cardiovascular and thrombotic risk factors. Venesection is used to reduce red cell numbers and low-dose aspirin as an anti-platelet agent. If these measures fail, cytoreductive therapies may be necessary.

Question 13

B Haemophilia A

Haemophilia A and B are both sex-linked recessive inherited diseases carried on the X chromosome. This means that males are affected but females remain carriers. Haemophilia A is caused by a deficiency of factor

VIII, while haemophilia B is caused by deficiency of factor IX. The disease may manifest once the child starts to mobilise and tumbles. From the blood results, we can see a normal platelet count, aggregation time and von Willebrand's factor (vWF) count. Factor VIII works in the intrinsic pathway of the coagulation mechanism and hence will affect the APTT time, not the thrombin or prothrombin times. Treatment can be to give factor VIII concentrate or desmopressin, which stimulates release of factor VIII by endothelial cells.

Question 14

B *Treatment dose low-molecular-weight heparin*
This lady is at high risk for developing a venous thromboembolism (VTE) and clinically sounds as though she has a left lower limb deep vein thrombosis (DVT). She has risk factors, including her age, recent orthopaedic surgery and has probably been immobile in hospital and at home following the procedure. There are no signs to suggest she is haemodynamically unstable or developed a PE. The diagnostic tests being arranged are likely to include Doppler scanning of the affected leg for a DVT and, if there is clinical concern, CT pulmonary angiography (CTPA) for a PE.

Given the risk of PE forming from a DVT she should be started on treatment. In the first instance this should be low-molecular-weight heparin at treatment dose. A prophylactic dose may have had a role to play in her admission and post operative discharge to reduce the risk of developing VTE but now she has signs to suggest a VTE she needs a treatment dose. There is no need to formally anticoagulate her with warfarin as the diagnosis needs to be confirmed. She may be converted to warfarin at a later stage of her treatment (currently recommended for 3–6 months depending on the clinical scenario). She is not clinically unstable so formal thrombolysis is not indicated.

VTE risk assessment is an important part of reducing a patient's chance of developing VTE either during their in-patient stay or in the weeks following. In-patients may receive specialist stockings or boots as mechanical thromboprophylaxis or chemical thromboprophylaxis with low-molecular-weight heparin at prophylactic doses.

Question 15

C *Result of massive blood transfusion*
The findings are in keeping with a massive blood transfusion. The low platelet count is most likely a dilutional thrombocytopenia (due to no platelets being

transfused concurrently and even being consumed in the surgical process). Blood given for transfusion contains no platelets due to the processing of different blood products from a donated sample.

The clotting times have all risen. Again this is partly explained by diluting the patient's serum (where clotting factors circulate) with transfused blood. Blood for transfusion contains hardly any serum and therefore no clotting factors due the fractionation post-donation. Additionally the diagnosis and surgery would have consumed clotting factors and these have yet to be replaced either physiologically or medically.

It is also likely she has an element of disseminated intravascular coagulopathy. Importantly she is clinically stable now and the patient's parameters should normalise naturally over a few days. If she deteriorates, further blood products such as platelets, plasma and so on would be necessary.

Question 16

D Disseminated intravascular coagulopathy

Disseminated intravascular coagulopathy (DIC) is caused by the release into the circulation of thromboplastin or another procoagulant which causes the blood to clot. Coagulation factors and platelets are consumed faster than they can be produced, resulting in haemorrhage. As the small clots consume coagulation proteins and platelets, normal coagulation is disrupted and abnormal bleeding occurs. The activation of the coagulation cascade forms thrombin that converts fibrinogen to fibrin. The fibrinolytic system then breaks down fibrinogen and fibrin, forming fibrin degradation products such as D-dimers. Fibrin strands in blood vessels damage red blood cells leading to the presence of fragmented cells on the blood film.

Common causes of DIC are sepsis, trauma, crush injuries, obstetric causes (amniotic fluid embolus, retroplacental haematoma) and malignancy. Despite the need for blood products to support the patient, the only effective treatment is reversal of the causative agent.

Question 17

B Lytic lesion

The hollowing of the bone is typical of a lytic lesion due to osteoclast dysregulation. The bone is hollowed and weak and thus prone to pathological process. Lytic lesions are a hallmark of myeloma although other malignant processes can mimic them.

Question 18

E *Myeloma*

Myeloma would be most likely, given the hallmark findings of bone pain, macrocytic anaemia, renal failure, raised serum protein (with a raised globulin count here of 52), urinary protein and hypercalcaemia.

Myeloma is an excess of plasma cells usually producing a paraprotein, hence the rise in globulin (and therefore total protein) and proteinuria (Bence–Jones protein).

Due to bone turnover it causes hypercalcaemia (which causes confusion) and bony pain and can lead to lytic lesions and pathological fractures, as in this case.

His urine dipstick is not typical of a urinary tract infection, although bacterial infections are common both in this age group and in myeloma, so microbiological testing would be performed. Although B12 deficiency can cause macrocytic anaemia and neurology, the other features would not be expected and the neuropathy is usually peripheral rather than central. A thorough drug history is necessary and NSAIDs may have been used and should be avoided given the renal failure (associated with myeloma).

This man needs hydration, analgesia and renal support. He needs further investigation, including skeletal survey (part shown in Question 17) and bone marrow examination. Treatment of myeloma involves chemotherapy, and in younger patients stem cell transplants are offered although relapse remains an issue whatever the treatment used.

Question 19

E *ALL*

This young girl's symptoms suggest she is anaemic and thrombocytopenic. This is confirmed by the blood tests but there is a very high WCC ('leukaemia'). She has no temperature, no rise in the neutrophils or C-reactive protein to suggest an infection although she is at very high risk of infection. The red spots are petechiae and not meningococcal sepsis.

Her blood film shows the high WCC is mostly due to immature white cells. There is a mature-looking neutrophil and the difference in size is appreciable.

She requires further investigation with bone marrow examination but the most likely diagnosis is ALL, which is the most common childhood malignancy. Once confirmed, she would be treated in a children's cancer centre with chemotherapy in the context of a clinical trial. Unlike other malignancies, the treatment is quite prolonged – 2 years in girls and 3 years in boys – although only the initial treatment and any complications are treated as in-patients.

Some patients are offered stem cell transplants. Even without this, the prognosis in children in excellent, whereas in adults it is quite poor.

Acute myeloid leukaemia is unusual in children (whereas in adults AML is much more common than ALL) and the blasts would be immature precursors to neutrophils with probably no normal neutrophils left. Treatment is again with chemotherapy and stem cell transplants if applicable.

The history is not typical for the chronic leukaemias. CML is rare in children occurring more in adolescence onwards. There is splenomegaly, usually quite pronounced, and often lymphadenopathy. The blood film and bone marrow would show an excess of myeloid white cells (everything but lymphocytes) and as a consequence anaemia and thrombocytopenia. CML is due to a change in the genetic structure causing the Philadelphia chromosome. Treatment has been revolutionised by tyrosine kinase inhibitors, leading to a good prognosis.

Chronic lymphocytic leukaemia is a disease of older adults. The patient may be completely asymptomatic with an incidental finding of excess mature lymphocytes on routine blood tests. Patients can develop other cytopenias and lymphadenopathy. Treatment is not always necessary but if indicated would include chemotherapy.

Question 20

1. C
2. B
3. A

This is a tricky question. To tackle it, one must be familiar with the different surface antigens on red blood cells (RBCs) and serum antibodies in the serum.

Blood group AB individuals have both A and B antigens on the surface of the RBCs but their blood serum does not contain any antibodies against either A or B antigen.

Blood group A individuals have the A antigen on the surface of their RBCs but their blood serum contains antibodies against the B antigen.

Blood group B individuals have the B antigen on the surface of their RBCs but their blood serum contains antibodies against the A antigen.

Blood group O individuals do not have either A or B antigens on the surface of their RBCs but their blood serum contains antibodies against the A and B blood group antigens.

Rh D+ patients are those who have D antigens on the surface of their RBCs.

4 Microbiology

Questions

Parveen Jayia and Hugo Donaldson

Question 1

A 68-year-old woman with a history of heavy alcohol use is admitted with signs of meningitis. The nurse on the ward looking after her informs you that the microbiology lab has phoned up and she has Gram-positive bacilli in her blood cultures.

Which of the following is the most likely organism in her cultures?

A. *Neisseria meningitidis*
B. *Haemophilus influenzae*
C. *Streptococcus pneumoniae*
D. *Listeria monocytogenes*
E. *Escherichia coli*

Question 2

You are asked to review a 42-year-old woman who developed a skin infection following a peripheral venous cannula insertion site infection 3 days ago. Microbiology phoned to tell you that her blood cultures have grown Gram-positive cocci. The nurse informs you the patient is known to be colonised with methicillin-resistant Staphylococcus aureus (MRSA).

Which of the following antibiotics is the most appropriate choice until sensitivities are known?

A. Meropenem
B. Vancomycin
C. Flucloxacillin
D. Clindamycin
E. Piperacillin/tazobactam (Tazocin)

Clinical Data Interpretation for Medical Finals: Single Best Answer Questions, First Edition.
Edited by Philip Socrates Pastides and Parveen Jayia.
© 2012 Philip Socrates Pastides and Parveen Jayia. Published 2012 by John Wiley & Sons, Ltd.

Question 3

You are asked to review an 83-year-old man who has just starting having profuse, foul-smelling green diarrhoea. He was admitted 7 days ago with a mild community-acquired pneumonia and has finished a 5-day course of clarithromycin. His white cell count (WCC) taken today has risen to $36 \times 10^9/L$, C-reactive protein (CRP) is 20 mg/L and his urea and creatinine have doubled compared with his admission bloods. On examination he is pyrexial, dehydrated and has mild diffuse abdominal tenderness.

What is the most appropriate next action?
A. PO metronidazole alone
B. PO metronidazole and IV vancomycin
C. IV metronidazole and PO vancomycin
D. IV vancomycin and urgent surgical review
E. IV metronidazole and PO vancomycin and urgent surgical review

Question 4

A 24-year-old student is admitted with a right lower lobar pneumonia, CURB score = 3. He is empirically commenced on IV co-amoxiclav 1.2 g tds plus IV clarithromycin 500 mg bd. His sputum culture report is as follows:
Streptococcus pneumoniae – isolated
Penicillin – I (intermediate) [minimum inhibitory concentration (MIC) = 0.5 mg/L]
Ceftriaxone – S (sensitive) (MIC = 0.25 mg/L)
Erythromycin – R (resistant)
Levofloxacin – S
Your consultant asks you to de-escalate his antibiotics once the sensitivities are known to the most narrow-spectrum effective agent.

Which of the following should you choose?
A. IV benzylpenicillin 1.2g qds
B. Iv co-amoxiclav 1.2 g tds
C. IV levofloxacin 500 mg bd
D. IV amoxicillin 1 g tds
E. IV vancomycin 1g bd

Question 5

You are reviewing a 53-year-old man with abnormal liver function tests. His hepatitis B serology is reported as follows:

Hepatitis B surface antigen (HBsAg) – negative
Total anti-HepB core antibody (Anti-HBc) – positive
Anti-HepB surface antibody (Anti-HBs) – positive

With which of the following scenarios are these results most consistent?
A. No evidence of current or past infection but in keeping with vaccination
B. Current infection with hepatitis B but not of recent onset
C. Past resolved hepatitis B infection
D. No evidence of current or past infection
E. Early acute infection with hepatitis B

Question 6

You are reviewing a 29-year-old pregnant woman's booking blood results. Her syphilis serology is shown below:
Syphilis total IgG/IgM – positive
Treponema pallidum particle agglutination (TPPA) – positive
Syphilis IgM – negative
Rapid plasma reagin (RPR) – negative

With which of the following scenarios are these results most consistent?
A. Active current syphilis infection
B. No evidence of syphilis infection at any time
C. Past successfully treated syphilis
D. Recent unsuccessfully treated syphilis
E. Indeterminate results; send to a reference laboratory for further testing

Question 7

A 76-year-old man has enterococcal endocarditis and is being treated with amoxicillin 2 g 4-hourly and gentamicin 60 mg 8-hourly. He has had peak and trough gentamicin levels sent before and after his third dose, the results of which are shown below:
Gentamicin post-dose (peak) level – 4 mg/L (3–5 mg/L)
Gentamicin pre-dose (trough) level – 2 mg/L (<1 mg/L)

How should you adjust his gentamicin dosing?
A. Leave his prescription as it is
B. Decrease the dose to 40 mg and keep the interval at 8-hourly
C. Stop his gentamicin
D. Decrease the dose to 40 mg and increase the interval to 24-hourly
E. Keep the dose at 60 mg but increase the interval to 12-hourly

Question 8

You are a GP seeing a 16-week pregnant woman who has been in contact with her niece who developed a non-vesicular rash. The patient is currently asymptomatic. Your colleague sends some serology and the following results are available:
Parvovirus B19 IgG – not detected
Parvovirus B19 IgM – not detected
Rubella IgG – detected
Rubella IgM – not detected
Measles IgG – detected
Measles IgM – not detected

What should you advise the patient?
A. Reassure her that she is immune to rubella and measles and has no evidence of infection with parvovirus B19 but ask her to return if she develops a rash. Reassure her that, as she is immune to rubella and measles and has no evidence of infection with parvovirus B19, the risk to the fetus is remote and no further action is needed.
B. Advise her that she is susceptible to parvovirus B19 and advise her to return in 1 month or if symptoms develop for repeat testing. Further management will depend on these results
C. Reassure her that she is immune to rubella and measles but advise her that she is susceptible to parvovirus B19 and offer her parvovirus B19 vaccination immediately
D. Reassure her that, as she is immune to rubella and measles and has no evidence of infection with parvovirus B19, the risk to the fetus is remote and no further action is needed
E. Reassure her that she is immune to rubella and measles but advise her that she is susceptible to parvovirus B19 and offer her parvovirus B19 vaccination after she has given birth

Question 9

You receive the following urine report on a sample sent from an 84-year-old woman in a nursing home.
WCC – $<10^4$/mL
Red cell count – not seen
Casts – not seen
Squamous epithelial cells – +++
Culture – *E. coli* $>10^5$ cfu/mL

With which of the following scenarios are these results most consistent?
A. A poorly taken sample with a high likelihood of contamination
B. Sterile pyuria
C. Significant bacterial growth in keeping with urinary tract infection which requires treatment regardless of the patient's symptoms
D. Chronic pyelonephritis with *E. coli*
E. Glomerulonephritis with a superimposed *E. coli* urinary tract infection

Question 10

A 69-year-old woman presents to your clinic with increased urinary frequency but no other symptoms. Urine dipstick results are shown below:
Nitrites – negative
Leucocytes – negative
Protein – negative
Blood – positive

Which of the following is the most appropriate course of action?
A. Strong evidence of bacterial urinary tract infection; commence antibiotics immediately
B. Strong evidence of bacterial urinary tract infection; send a midstream sample of urine and then commence antibiotics
C. Strong evidence of bacterial urinary tract infection; send a midstream sample of urine but wait for results before commencing antibiotics
D. No strong evidence of infection; consider other diagnoses
E. No strong evidence of infection on dipstick; however, in view of symptoms commence antibiotics anyway

Question 11

You are asked to review a 32-year-old man in A&E who has presented with a fever of 38.2°C and a headache. His flatmate brought him to A&E as she felt he has been confused for the past day. She says he has no significant past medical history. A CT scan has been preliminarily reported as normal. His cerebrospinal fluid report is as follows:

Appearance – clear and colourless fluid

WCC – 120 × 10⁶/L (90% lymphocytes)

Red cell count – 10 × 10⁶/L

Gram stain – no organisms seen

CSF protein – 0.6 g/L (0.2–0.4)

CSF glucose – 3.6 mmol/L

Serum glucose – 5.2 mmol/L

Which of the following organisms is the most likely cause of his symptoms?

A. *Neisseria meningitidis*

B. *Mycobacterium tuberculosis*

C. *Streptococcus pneumoniae*

D. *Listeria monocytogenes*

E. Herpes simplex

Question 12

You are reviewing a 57-year-old homeless woman in your surgery. She has been complaining of a persistent cough, night sweats and weight loss. She had failed to attend previous appointments but your colleague previously arranged a chest X-ray which shows a patchy infiltrate in the right upper lobe. Sputum sent at the same time is reported as follows:

Normal upper respiratory flora +++

S. aureus sensitive to flucloxacillin and clarithromycin

Auramine stain no acid- and alcohol-fast bacilli seen

Mycobacterium species not isolated

Which of the following is the most appropriate next course of action?

A. Refer urgently to local TB services

B. TB ruled out, send urine for pneumococcal and Legionella urinary antigens

C. Commence TB therapy with rifampicin, isoniazid, pyrazinamide and ethambutol

D. TB ruled out, send serum for mycoplasma, Q fever and chlamydia serology

E. TB ruled out, commence flucloxacillin

Question 13

Which of the following conditions is NOT notifiable in England and Wales?

A. Leptospirosis
B. Brucellosis
C. Acute encephalitis
D. Acute meningitis
E. Malaria

Question 14

A patient with a chronic venous leg ulcer has been attending the dressing clinic. He has a swab of his ulcer sent, the results of which are shown below. On questioning the nurse who dressed the wound she states that it looked sloughy with some serous exudate but otherwise appears to be improving.
Proteus spp.+ sensitive: co-amoxiclav, ciprofloxacin, cefuroxime; resistant: amoxicillin
E. coli ++ sensitive: co-amoxiclav, ciprofloxacin, cefuroxime; resistant: amoxicillin
Coagulase-negative stapylococci +

Which of the following is the most appropriate next course of action?

A. Commence PO co-amoxiclav
B. Commence PO ciprofloxacin
C. Refer to hospital for IV co-amoxiclav
D. Do not start antibiotics and ask the nurse not to re-swab the wound unless there is clinical evidence of infection
E. Do not start antibiotics and but ask the nurse to re-swab the wound the next time she dresses it.

Question 15

While you are on call the microbiology laboratory telephones with a blood culture result. The aerobic bottle has grown Gram-positive cocci in chains.

With which of the following organisms are these results most consistent?

A. *Staphylococcus aureus*
B. *Streptococcus pyogenes* (group A streptococci)
C. *Neisseria meningitidis*
D. *Bacillus cereus*
E. *Escherichia coli*

Question 16

The microbiology laboratory telephones and states that your patient's blood cultures have grown Streptococcus gallolyticus (Streptococcus bovis group).

With which of the following clinical conditions are these streptococci particularly associated?

A. Adenocarcinoma of the colon and endocarditis
B. Necrotising fasciitis
C. Pneumonia and meningitis
D. 'Viridans' streptococci, oral commensals of low pathogenic potential
E. Pyogenic abscess formation

Question 17

You are reviewing a 45-year-old patient who returned from holiday in Portugal 2 days ago. She was admitted with community-acquired pneumonia and some of her results are back, as follows:
Legionella urinary antigen: negative
Mycoplasma pneumoniae complement fixation test: <1:10
Q fever complement fixation test: <1:10
Chlamydophilia pneumoniae complement fixation test: <1:10

Which of the following is the most appropriate course of action?

A. Legionella infection ruled out but infection with other organisms not excluded; send repeat serology for *M. pneumoniae*, Q fever and *C. pneumoniae*.
B. Infection with Legionella, *M. pneumoniae*, Q fever and *C. pneumoniae* excluded; no further tests should be sent
C. Infection with *M. pneumoniae*, Q fever and *C. pneumoniae* excluded; send Legionella serology and culture samples
D. Insufficient evidence to exclude infection with any of the tested organisms; send Legionella serology and culture samples and repeat serology for the other organisms

E. Insufficient evidence to exclude infection with any of the tested organisms; repeat Legionella urinary antigen and repeat serology for the other organisms.

Question 18

You are reviewing a 71-year-old woman 72 hours post-colectomy for rectal carcinoma. She is apyrexial and has no chest signs or symptoms. Her pulse rate is 72 beats/min, her blood pressure is 132/78 mmHg, and her O_2 saturation by pulse oximetry is 94% on room air.

Sputum cultures have grown Klebsiella pneumoniae +++ sensitive to co-amoxiclav, cefuroxime, ciprofloxacin and piperacillin/tazobactam.

What is the most appropriate antibiotic regime?

A. Commence IV piperacillin/tazobactam
B. Do not commence any antibiotics
C. Commence PO co-amoxiclav
D. Commence PO ciprofloxacin
E. Commence IV cefuroxime and metronidazole

Question 19

You are reviewing a 67-year-old man who had a prosthetic hip replacement 5 months ago. He has now presented with progressively increasing joint pain but has been apyrexial with no local swelling or erythema. He had an arthroscopy performed and fluid and tissue samples sent prior to antibiotics to look for evidence of infection. The results are as follows:

- Fluid 1: microscopy – white cells not seen, no organisms seen, culture: *Bacillus* spp. isolated on enrichment only
- Fluid 2: microscopy – white cells not seen, no organisms seen, culture: no growth after 7 days
- Tissue 1: microscopy – white cells not seen, no organisms seen, culture: no growth after 7 days
- Tissue 2: microscopy – white cells not seen, no organisms seen, culture: coagulase-negative staphylococci isolated on enrichment only
- Tissue 3: microscopy – white cells not seen, no organisms seen, culture: no growth after 7 days

How would you interpret these results?

A. Evidence of infection with *Bacillus* spp. and coagulase-negative staphylococci

B. Evidence of infection with *Bacillus* spp.; coagulase-negative staphylococci are skin commensals of low pathogenic potential and likely to be contaminants

C. Evidence of infection with coagulase-negative staphylococci; *Bacillus* spp. are skin commensals of low pathogenic potential and likely to be contaminants

D. No definitive evidence of infection on these results alone; correlate with clinical, histological and radiological findings

E. Evidence of infection with an organism other than coagulase-negative staphylococci and *Bacillus* spp., which are skin commensals of low pathogenic potential and likely to be contaminants. Causative organism may be something else

Question 20

A 49-year-old man has been admitted to your ward with a clinical diagnosis of pyelonephritis. The referring GP letter states he is colonised with an extended spectrum beta-lactamase (ESBL) producing E. coli but no sensitivities are provided and the result isn't on the hospital's laboratory system. The patient is tachycardic, hypotensive and has had a rigor. You take blood and urine cultures and then commence antibiotics.

Which of the following antibiotics is most likely to have activity against the organism and should be commenced?

A. Ciprofloxacin

B. Ceftriaxone

C. Ertapenem

D. Piperacillin/tazobactam (Tazocin)

E. Gentamicin

Microbiology

Answers

Question 1

D Listeria monocytogenes

Listeria monocytogenes is a Gram-positive bacillus. *Neisseria meningitidis* and *Haemophilus influenzae* are Gram-negative cocci with *Neisseria meningitidis* usually in pairs (diplococci). *Streptococcus pneumoniae* is a Gram-positive coccus often in pairs or short chains. *Escherichia coli* is a Gram-negative bacillus.

Listeria monocytogenes is inherently resistant to ceftriaxone and cefotaxime but is sensitive to amoxicillin. Neonates, immunosuppressed patients and patients over 55 years old are at increased risk of *Listeria* infections and amoxicillin should be included in any empirical regime

Question 2

B Vancomycin

Vancomycin is a glycopeptide antibiotic active against most Gram-positive organisms and resistance is rare. It is the treatment of choice for MRSA bacteraemia.

Meropenem, flucloxacillin and piperacillin/tazobactam are all ß-lactam antibiotics which have activity against methicillin-sensitive *Staphylococcus aureus* (MSSA) *however,* MRSA has an altered penicillin binding protein (PBP2a) and is inherently resistant to all ß-lactam antibiotics.

Most of the common hospital acquired strains of MRSA in the UK are resistant to erythromycin, clindamycin and ciprofloxacin although many community acquired strains are sensitive to these antibiotics.

Question 3

E IV metronidazole and PO vancomycin and urgent surgical review

This patient has signs and symptoms suggestive of severe *Clostridium difficile* infection (CDI). CDI has been particularly associated with third-generation cephalosporins, clindamycin and ciprofloxacin, but can occur with almost any antibiotic and should be considered in any patient with diarrhoea following a course of antibiotics. IV vancomycin is not useful in the treatment of CDI.

The current best practice guidance: '*Clostridium difficile* infection: How to deal with the problem', was published by the Department of Health and Health Protection Agency in December 2008.

It recommends the using the following as markers of severe CDI:

- WCC > 15×10^9/L
- acutely rising blood creatinine (e.g. >50% increase above baseline)
- temperature >38.5 °C
- evidence of severe colitis (abdominal signs, radiology).

For the treatment of life-threatening CDI, consult your local hospital policy; however, the national guidance recommends: oral vancomycin up to 500 mg qds for 10–14 days via nasogastric tube or rectal installation plus IV metronidazole 500 mg tds. Such patients should be closely monitored, with specialist surgical input, and should have their blood lactate measured. Colectomy should be considered, especially if caecal dilatation is >10 cm. Colectomy is best performed before blood lactate rises > 5 mmol/L, when survival is extremely poor.

Question 4

A IV benzylpenicillin 1.2 g qds
Streptococcus pneumoniae isolates with an MIC $\leq$ 2 mg/L are considered susceptible to β-lactam agents except in infections of the central nervous system (CNS). Penicillin resistance is due to alterations in the penicillin-binding proteins, however high-level resistance is rare in the UK. Intermediate resistance such as in this case can be overcome with higher doses of β-lactam agents, with CNS infections being the exception.

All of the other agents listed could be used but they all have a broader spectrum of activity than benzylpenicillin.

The clavulanic acid component of co-amoxiclav is a β-lactamase inhibitor; however, as β-lactamase production is not the mechanism of resistance in this case it is not required. Amoxicillin is a broad-spectrum penicillin with more Gram-negative activity than benzylpenicillin. Vancomycin is recommended for high-level penicillin-resistant isolates or CNS infection but in this case is not required.

Levofloxacin has modest activity against pneumococci *in vitro*; however, the British Thoracic Society recommends combining it with another agent active against *S. pneumoniae* such as IV benzylpenicillin when managing high-severity community-acquired pneumonia ('BTS guidelines for the management of community acquired pneumonia in adults: update 2009'. *Thorax* 2009; 64(Suppl III): iii1–iii55).

Question 5

C *Past resolved hepatitis B infection*
Most laboratories will test HBsAg to look for evidence of current infection and HepB surface antibody titre post-vaccination to assess immunity. Following vaccination but without a history of previous infection, the anti-HBc result would be negative.

If the HBsAg is positive then further serology will be carried out to clarify whether it is consistent with acute or chronic infection. It is good practice to repeat a positive test immediately to confirm the patient's identity and the result.

Question 6

C *Past successfully treated syphilis*
Total IgG/IgM is commonly used as a screening test and, if positive, further tests are then undertaken. A specific treponemal test, e.g. TPPA, is indicative of a treponemal infection either currently or at some time in the past. Once these tests have become positive, their usefulness is limited because they can remain positive for life. A non-treponemal antibody test, e.g. RPR, is useful for monitoring treatment. The failure of the RPR titre to fall more than fourfold or become negative suggests a persistent infection, reinfection or a false-positive test. The RPR titre is at it's highest during the secondary and early latent stages of syphilis and declines thereafter.

In this case the results are also in keeping with untreated syphilis in the past. With an RPR which has declined to undetectable levels, the past medical history of the patient is important in interpreting these results.

It is good practice to repeat a positive test immediately to confirm the patient's identity and the result.

Question 7

E *Keep the dose at 60 mg but increase the interval to 12-hourly*
A pre-dose level is useful for monitoring any accumulation of the drug which could be associated with toxicity. In this case, the elevated pre-dose level suggests that the drug is being given too frequently for this patient. A post-dose level is useful for ensuring enough of the drug is being given. In this case the level is within the recommended therapeutic range for this

indication so the dose of drug need not be adjusted. A low post-dose level suggests too low a dose of drug is being given and a high post-dose level suggests too high a dose of drug is being given. Option risks giving too little of the drug. Always refer to local protocols and liaise with the pharmacy department if required.

(T. S. J. Elliott *et al.* Guidelines for the antibiotic treatment of endocarditis in adults: report of the Working Party of the British Society for Antimicrobial Chemotherapy. *Journal of Antimicrobial Chemotherapy* 2004; 54: 971–981.)

Question 8

B *Advise her that she is susceptible to parvovirus B19 and advise her to return in 1 month or if symptoms develop for repeat testing. Further management will depend on these results*

This patient is immune to measles and rubella as shown by the positive IgG results. She is susceptible to parvovirus B19 and it may be too early in the course of infection for her to have seroconverted. Infection within the first 20 weeks of pregnancy is associated with hydrops fetalis which has a mortality of approx. 50% if untreated. Maternal asymptomatic parvovirus B19 infection is at least as likely to infect and damage the fetus as symptomatic infection, so the patient should be tested 1 month after exposure to see if she has seroconverted, whether she has been symptomatic or not. If the repeat serology is suggestive of parvovirus B19 infection, specialist advice should be sought. There is no parvovirus B19 vaccine currently available.

The publication 'Guidance on viral rash in pregnancy' (Health Protection Agency, January 2011) gives detail on the management of rash and contact with rash in pregnancy.

Question 9

A *A poorly taken sample with a high likelihood of contamination*

In most cases, urine culture should be interpreted with regard to the clinical picture, presence or absence of white cells (which are associated with infection) and squamous epithelial cells (indicative of contamination). There are some exceptions to this, such as asymptomatic bacteriuria in pregnancy, which should always be treated, as it is associated with pyelonephritis and early delivery.

In the absence of symptoms this patient should not be commenced on antibiotics.

The Health Protection Agency document 'Diagnosis of UTI quick reference guide for primary care' gives more information and current national recommendations.

Question 10

D *No strong evidence of infection; consider other diagnoses*
Urine nitrite is formed when bacteria reduce the nitrate that is normally present. Leucocyte esterase detects intact and lysed leucocytes produced in inflammation. The presence of nitrites and leucocytes is suggestive of bacterial urinary tract infection (UTI). If both are negative, UTI is unlikely. Haematuria and proteinuria both occur in UTI but they also occur in other conditions and in this case the absence of nitrites, leucocytes or severe symptoms suggests UTI is unlikely.

The Health Protection Agency document 'Diagnosis of UTI quick reference guide for primary care' gives more information and current national recommendations.

Question 11

E *Herpes simplex*
The normal CSF glucose level ≥60% of simultaneously determined plasma concentration suggests a viral rather than a bacterial cause. In bacterial meningitis, the CSF WCC is typically raised and predominantly polymorphs. The protein level is elevated and the serum glucose level decreased to <60% of simultaneously determined plasma concentration.

In tuberculous meningitis the white cells are usually lymphocytes, the protein is elevated and the glucose decreased. The presence of polymorphs or lymphocytes must be interpreted with caution as viral and tuberculous meningitis may be associated with polymorphs rather than lymphocytes early in the infection.

(Health Protection Agency (2008). *Investigation of cerebrospinal fluid*. National Standard Method BSOP 27 Issue 5.)

Question 12

A *Refer urgently to local TB services*
This patient has chest X-ray signs and symptoms suggestive of pulmonary tuberculosis. One negative sputum stain and culture result does not rule out pulmonary tuberculosis, especially if the clinical suspicion is high.

Current NICE guidance on the diagnosis of active respiratory TB recommends the following:

- a posterior–anterior chest X-ray; chest X-ray appearances suggestive of TB should lead to further diagnostic investigation
- multiple sputum samples (at least three, with one early morning sample) should be sent for TB microscopy and culture before starting treatment if possible or, failing that, within 7 days of starting.

NICE Clinical Guideline 33. 'Tuberculosis: clinical diagnosis and management of tuberculosis, and measures for its prevention and control'.

Tuberculosis should always be managed by a specialist in tuberculosis treatment and a referral to the local TB services should be made in this case.

Question 13

A *Leptospirosis*

Notification of certain infectious diseases to the relevant local public health authorities is an important role. Notification prompts local investigation and appropriate action to control the specified disease. Under the Health Protection (Notification) Regulations 2010, doctors in England and Wales have a statutory duty to notify a 'proper officer' of the local authority of suspected cases of certain infectious diseases. A notification certificate should be completed immediately on diagnosis of a suspected notifiable disease and you should not wait for laboratory confirmation of the suspected infection or contamination before notification.

It is important to be aware of local notification arrangements and which conditions require notification. A current list of notifiable diseases can be found at: www.hpa.org.uk/Topics/InfectiousDiseases/InfectionsAZ/NotificationsOfInfectiousDiseases/ListOfNotifiableDiseases/

Question 14

D *Do not start antibiotics and ask the nurse not to re-swab the wound unless there is clinical evidence of infection*

Microbial contamination of leg ulcers is universal and a positive microbiology sample cannot be used to determine the presence of infection in a leg ulcer, as this is a clinical diagnosis. Sending swabs routinely for bacteriology is therefore of no benefit. Clinical evidence of infection, such as pain, erythema, oedema, fever and cellulitis, should be sought. A sample should be sent for culture prior to commencing treatment on clinical grounds to determine the organisms present and their antimicrobial sensitivities.

The fact that sensitivities are reported does not mean that treatment is recommended.

Question 15

B *Streptococcus pyogenes (group A Streptococci)*
Streptococci are Gram-positive cocci and are usually arranged in chains. Some streptococci such as *Streptococcus pneumoniae* and enterococci may been in short pairs and chains. Staphylococci are also Gram-positive cocci but they are usually arranged in clumps. *Neisseria meningitidis* are Gram-negative cocci usually in pairs (diplococci). *Bacillus* spp. are Gram-positive bacilli (rods) and E. coli are Gram-negative bacilli.

Question 16

A *Adenocarcinoma of the colon and endocarditis oral commensals of low pathogenic potential*
Streptococcus bovis bacteraemia has a high correlation with gastrointestinal malignancy, particularly of the colon and endocarditis. Patients with *S. bovis* bacteraemia should be investigated for colonic malignancy. *S. gallolyticus* and *S. pasteurianus* are the two members of the *S. bovis* group most associated with malignancy and clinicians should be aware of the nomenclature. Group A streptococci (*S. pyogenes*) are associated with necrotising fasciitis.

Streptococcus pneumoniae is associated with pneumonia and meningitis. The *S. milleri* group (*S. intermedius, S. constellatus, S. anginosus*) is associated with abscess formation.

(Health Protection Agency (2007). Identification of Streptococcus species, Enterococcus species and morphologically similar organisms. National Standard Method BSOP ID 4 Issue 2.1.)

Question 17

D *Insufficient evidence to exclude infection with any of the tested organisms; send Legionella serology and culture samples and repeat serology for the other organisms*
The complement fixation test is a serology test. Response to infection may be demonstrated by the development of, or increase in the levels of, a specific antibody to the causative agent between two specimens; one taken in the acute phase of illness and the other taken in the convalescent phase.

In this case, only one sample has been sent so infection cannot be ruled out yet. A repeat sample should be sent to look for a rise in titre.

Legionella urinary antigen kits may only look for serogroup 1. This serogroup is associated with about 80% of infections but other serogroups may be involved. Clinicians should be aware that a negative Legionella urinary antigen result does not rule out Legionella infection. If infection with Legionella is suspected clinically, specimens should be sent for culture and serology.

Question 18

B *Do not commence any antibiotics*
Enterobacteriaceae, especially *Klebsiella* spp., *E. coli* and *Enterobacter* spp. along with *P. aeruginosa* and *S. aureus* are the most common organisms isolated from respiratory specimens of patients known or suspected to have hospital-acquired pneumonia

However, not all organisms isolated from respiratory specimens should be regarded as pathogens that necessarily require therapy. As with all microbiology results they should be interpreted and treated if necessary in the light of the full clinical picture. This patient has no clinical evidence of pneumonia at present, and commencing unnecessary antibiotics will put her at increased risk of adverse effects such as *C. difficile*-associated diarrhoea.

The clinical diagnosis of hospital-acquired pneumonia is difficult and there are no universally accepted clinical criteria. The British Society for Antimicrobial Chemotherapy recommends the following criteria to identify patients in whom pneumonia should be considered in the differential diagnosis:

1. Purulent tracheal secretions, and new and/or persistent infiltrate on chest X-ray, which is otherwise unexplained
2. Increased oxygen requirement
3. Core temperature >38.3 °C
4. Blood leucocytosis (>10 000/mm^3) or leucopenia (<4000/mm^3).

(R. G. Masterton *et al.* Guidelines for the management of hospital-acquired pneumonia in the UK. Journal of Antimicrobial Chemotherapy 2008; 62: 5–34.)

Question 19

D *No definitive evidence of infection on these results alone; correlate with clinical, histological and radiological findings*
The diagnosis of prosthetic joint infection is complex and specialist advice should be sought early. A review in the BMJ gives a good overview of the issues but generally multiple samples should be sent for culture and histopathology. The isolation of the same organism from two culture samples is in keeping

with infection, although for more virulent organisms such as *S. aureus* one positive culture is often accepted as confirming the diagnosis.

In this case, two different organisms have been isolated from enrichment only, which implies they were present in small numbers. The presence of white cells would also be suggestive of infection. In this case correlation should be made with clinical, histological and radiological findings, and a definitive surgical strategy and antibiotic regimen made on the basis of the results of these investigations.

(Philippa C. Matthews *et al.* Diagnosis and management of prosthetic joint infection *BMJ* 2009; 338: b1773.)

Question 20

C Ertapenem

Extended spectrum beta-lactamase-producing organisms are important because they are resistant to cephalosporins (cefuroxime, ceftriaxone, ceftazidime) often given as first-line agents to many severely ill patients. Many ESBL producers are multi-resistant to other groups of antibiotics such as ciprofloxacin, aminoglycosides(gentamicin, amikacin) and trimethoprim, narrowing treatment options. Sensitivities of ESBL producers to β-lactamase inhibitor combinations (piperacillin/tazobactam, co-amoxiclav) vary with the strain. Treatment outcome for β-lactamase inhibitor combinations appears to be unpredictable, particularly for severe infections. Carbapenems (imipenem, meropenem and ertapenem) are active against ESBL producers, and in this case a carbapenem should be used initially, as the patient is severely unwell. This may be de-escalated to a narrower-spectrum agent once sensitivities become available. Further information can be found in Health Protection Agency (2008). 'Laboratory detection and reporting of bacteria with extended spectrum β-lactamases'. National Standard Method, QSOP 51, Issue 2.2.

5 Radiology

Questions

Prasanna L. Perera and Vimal Raj

Question 1

A generally fit 30-year-old woman presents with sudden onset severe occipital headache. She has never experienced such symptoms before and on examination appears to have photophobia. A CT brain is requested and a representative image is shown below:

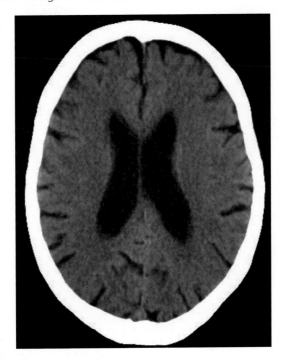

Clinical Data Interpretation for Medical Finals: Single Best Answer Questions, First Edition.
Edited by Philip Socrates Pastides and Parveen Jayia.
© 2012 Philip Socrates Pastides and Parveen Jayia. Published 2012 by John Wiley & Sons, Ltd.

What is the next appropriate investigation to confirm clinical suspicion?
A. Visual acuity testing
B. Chest radiography
C. Electroencephalography (EEG)
D. Cerebral angiography
E. Lumbar puncture

Question 2

A 45-year-old homeless man with a known history of alcohol abuse presents with a vague history of falls, confusion, drowsiness and a Glasgow Coma Score (GCS) of 12. A CT brain was performed and is shown below:

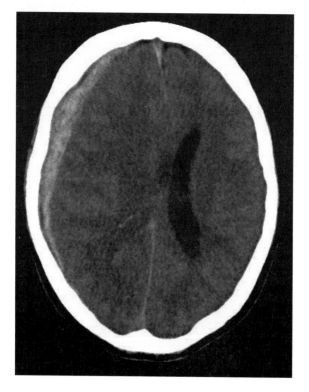

What is the appropriate treatment?

A. Watch and wait
B. Right cranial burr hole and evacuation of haematoma
C. Left craniotomy
D. Right craniotomy
E. Thrombolysis

Question 3

A 19-year-old rugby player is admitted with a history of headaches, vomiting, drowsiness and confusion 6 hours after a game during which he suffered a head injury. His CT scan is shown below:

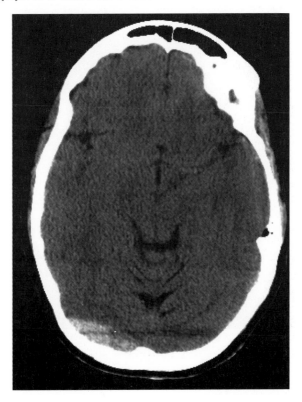

What does the CT show?

A. Subarachnoid haemorrhage

B. Infarct

C. Subdural haemorrhage

D. Tumour

E. Extradural haemorrhage

Question 4

A 70-year-old hypertensive woman is brought into A&E having been found unconscious at home. Her CT scan is shown below:

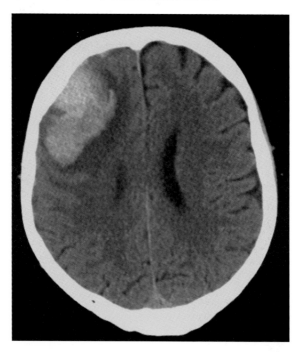

What does the CT show?

A. Intracerebral haemorrhage

B. Subdural haemorrhage

C. Multiple sclerosis

D. Infarct

E. Subarachnoid haemorrhage

Question 5

A 68-year-old man whose CT is shown below presented with weakness and speech disturbance.

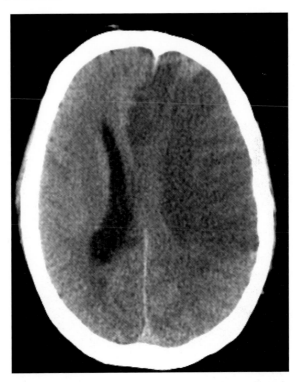

What does the CT show?
A. Intracerebral haemorrhage
B. Infarction
C. Multiple sclerosis
D. Tumour
E. Abscess

Question 6

A 22-year-old, generally fit man presents with sudden onset right pleuritic chest pain and dyspnoea. A chest X-ray is taken (below).

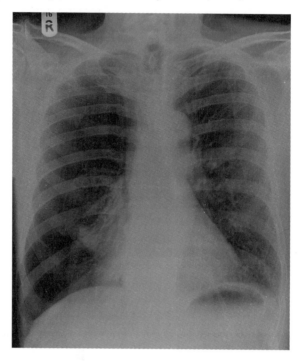

What does the chest X-ray show?

A. Infection
B. Pulmonary oedema
C. Pneumothorax
D. Pulmonary embolus
E. Impacted foreign body

Question 7

A 65-year-old man presents with a history of worsening abdominal pain and distension. On examination he is tachycardic and tachypnoeic. He is tender to palpation in the epigastric region. An erect chest X-ray is performed and is shown below:

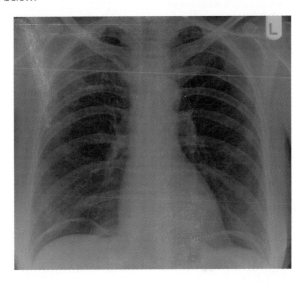

Based on the chest X-ray what is the most appropriate definitive management?

A. Nasogastric (NG) tube insertion

B. Laparotomy

C. CT of the chest and abdomen

D. Urinary catheter insertion

E. Admission to intensive care unit

Question 8

A 70-year-old woman presents with weight loss and shortness of breath. Her chest X-ray is shown below:

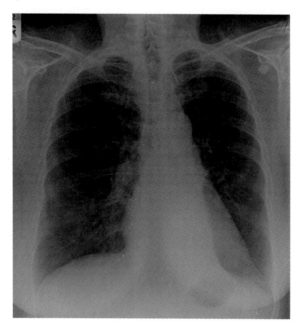

What does the chest X-ray show?

A. Pulmonary oedema
B. Left upper lobe collapse
C. Pneumothorax
D. Left lower lobe collapse
E. Rib fracture

Question 9

A 70-year-old man presents with cough and shortness of breath. His chest X-ray is shown below:

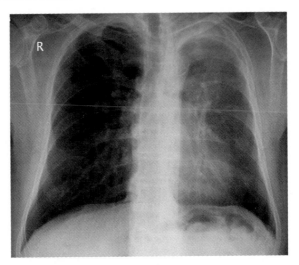

What does the chest X-ray show?
A. Lingular collapse
B. Consolidation
C. Left lower lobe collapse
D. Left upper lobe collapse
E. Pulmonary oedema

Question 10

A 65-year-old woman presents with a persistent cough. Her chest X-ray is shown below:

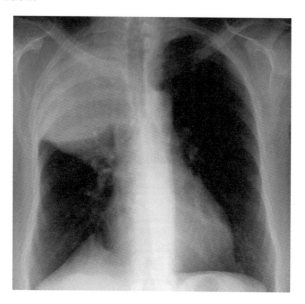

What does the chest X-ray show?

A. Pneumothorax
B. Pulmonary embolus
C. Right middle lobe collapse
D. Right upper lobe collapse
E. Left ventricular failure

Question 11

A 63-year-old woman present with a persistent productive cough. Her chest X-ray is shown below:

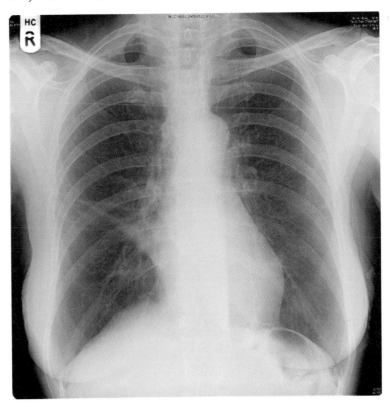

What does the chest X-ray show?
A. Right middle lobe collapse
B. Pneumothorax
C. Pulmonary embolus
D. Right upper lobe collapse
E. Right lower lobe collapse

Question 12

A 60-year-old man presents with acute shortness of breath. His chest X-ray is shown below:

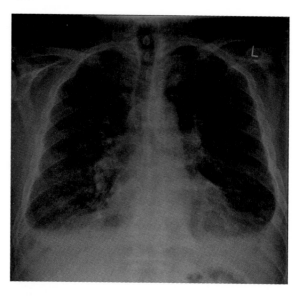

What treatment does he require?
A. Diuretics
B. Anticoagulation
C. Antibiotics
D. Surgical referral
E. Aspiration

Question 13

A 55-year-old woman presents with SOB and weight loss. Her chest X-ray is shown below:

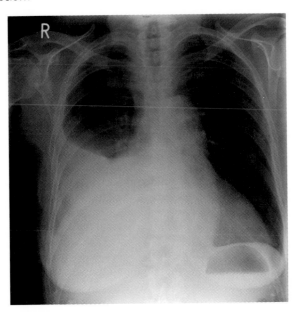

What does the chest X-ray show?
A. Pulmonary embolus
B. Pulmonary oedema
C. Right pleural effusion
D. Right consolidation
E. Tumour

Question 14

A 45-year-old women presents with fever, rigors and a cough productive of sputum. Her chest X-ray is shown below:

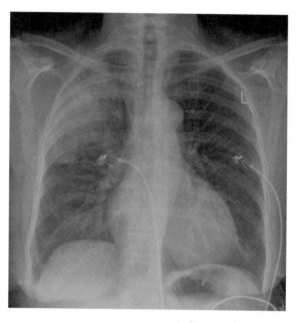

What is the most appropriate treatment?
A. Chest drain
B. Antibiotics
C. Diuretics
D. NG tube
E. Watch and wait

Question 15

A 70-year-old smoker presents with shortness of breath and weight loss. His chest X-ray is shown below:

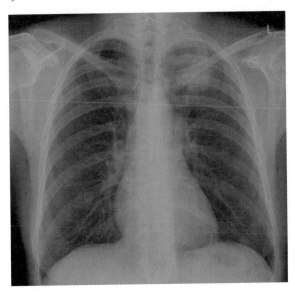

What does the chest X-ray show?

A. Left apical mass
B. Lingular collapse
C. Left pneumothorax
D. Pulmonary embolus
E. Pulmonary oedema

Question 16

Consider the X-ray below:

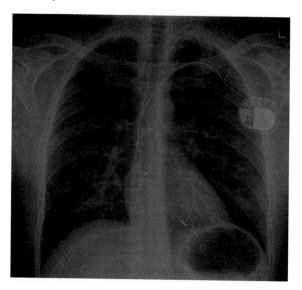

What underlying condition is this patient likely to have?

A. Pulmonary oedema
B. Angina
C. Cardiac arrhythmia
D. Tumour
E. Pneumothorax

Question 17

A 2-year-old boy is brought to A&E by his mother for difficulty in breathing. He was left unattended by his parents for 2 hours prior to the presentation. On examination, he has stridor but is afebrile. His chest X-ray is shown below:

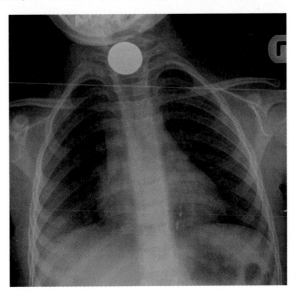

What is the most likely diagnosis?

A. Lung cancer
B. Infection
C. Swallowed foreign body
D. Hiatus hernia
E. Meningitis

Question 18

A 40-year-old woman presents with chest pain and shortness of breath. A CT scan (below) is performed after initial investigations.

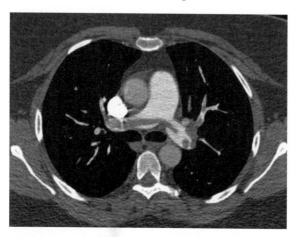

What treatment does the patient require?

A. Thoracocentesis
B. Antibiotics
C. Chest drain
D. Anticoagulation
E. Diuretics

Question 19

A 70-year-old woman presents with increasing abdominal pain and vomiting. Her past medical history includes bilateral inguinal hernia repair. On examination, the abdomen is distended but not tender. An abdominal radiograph was performed and is shown below:

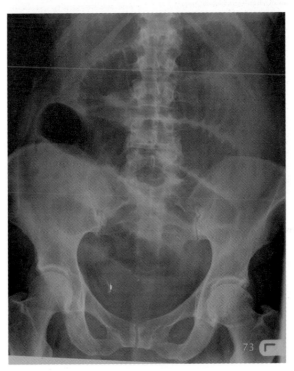

What is the diagnosis?

A. Pneumoperitoneum
B. Small bowel obstruction
C. Large bowel obstruction
D. Foreign body
E. Gallstones

Question 20

A 55-year-old woman presents with abdominal pain. Her abdominal X-ray is shown below:

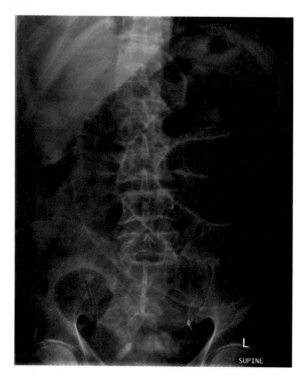

What does the abdominal X-ray show?

A. Large bowel obstruction
B. Colitis
C. Pneumoperitoneum
D. Gall stone
E. Renal calculus

Question 21

A 70-year-old man presents with abdominal pain and vomiting. His abdominal X-ray is shown below:

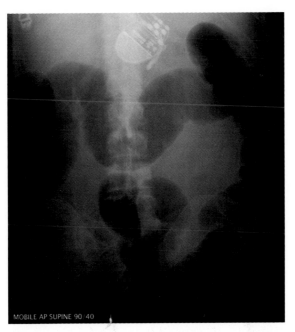

MOBILE AP SUPINE 90/40

What does his abdominal X-ray show?
A. Pneumoperitoneum
B. Small bowel obstruction
C. Large bowel obstruction
D. Foreign body
E. Gallstones

Question 22

A 35-year-old woman presents with chronic abdominal pain. Her abdominal X-ray is shown below:

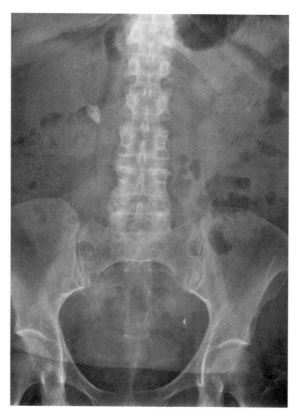

What does her abdominal X-ray show?
A. Colitis
B. Gallstones
C. Pneumoperitoneum
D. Renal calculi
E. Hip fracture

Question 23

A 60-year-old woman presents with abdominal pain and nausea. Her abdominal X-ray is shown below:

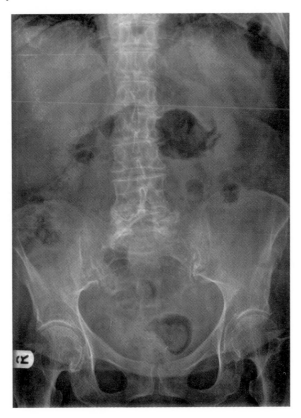

What does her abdominal X-ray show?

A. Ascites
B. Renal calculi
C. Pneumoperitoneum
D. Colitis
E. Gallstones

Question 24

A 70-year-old man presents to A&E with increasing right loin pain radiating to the groin. He denies any history of haematuria or dysuria. On examination, he is tachycardic but his blood pressure is maintained. A CT of the abdomen is performed (representative slice shown below) to assess him further.

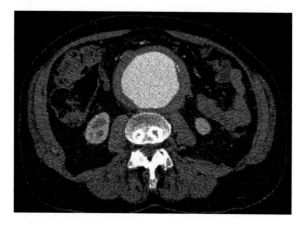

What is the most appropriate management?
A. Discharge him home
B. Refer him to the urologist for a possible renal stone
C. Refer him to the surgical team
D. Start anticoagulation
E. Organise MRI of the abdomen

Question 25

An 80-year-old woman undergoes a barium enema examination for contin-ued weight loss and altered bowel habits. A representative image from the examination is shown below:

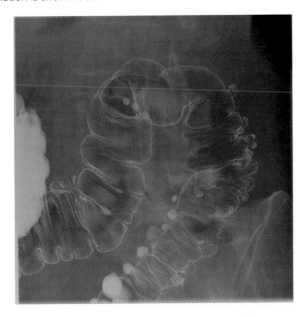

What is the diagnosis?

A. Diverticular disease
B. Large bowel obstruction
C. Pseudo-membranous colitis
D. Benign stricture
E. Malignant colorectal disease

Question 26

An 80-year-old woman underwent a barium enema examination for continued weight loss and altered bowel habits. A representative image from the examination is shown below:

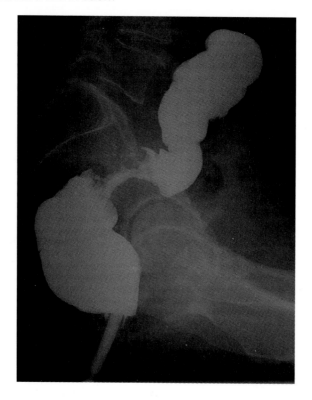

What is the diagnosis?
A. Mild diverticulitis
B. Severe diverticulitis
C. Pseudo-membranous colitis
D. Large bowel obstruction
E. Malignant colorectal disease

Radiology

Answers

Question 1

E *Lumbar puncture*
The history given represents a typical presentation of subarachnoid haemor-rhage (SAH). The CT image does not show any signs of haemorrhage or raised intracranial pressure.

Signs of a SAH include high attenuation (blood) in the sulci and basal cisterns. It is important to look for consequent mass effect, hydrocephalus and herniation. In cases of traumatic SAH, there may be associated fractures or subdural haemorrhages.

The commonest cause of SAH is trauma. The most common cause of a non-traumatic SAH is rupture of a Berry aneurysm in a cerebral artery. In 5% of patients with SAH, CT can be negative and clinical suspicion should be confirmed by a lumbar puncture.

Question 2

B *Right cranial burr hole and evacuation of haematoma*
A crescentic collection is seen over the cerebral hemisphere with displacement of the adjacent brain and compressed sulci medially in keeping with subdural haematoma (SDH).

Appropriate management of acute SDH is a cranial burr hole with evac-uation of the haematoma. Thrombolysis is only used in patients thought to have an embolic event such as infarction.

A history of falls, fluctuating levels of consciousness and headaches should alert the clinician to the possibility of a SDH. Alcoholics and elderly patients are particularly vulnerable. Bleeding occurs from rupture of bridging veins in the subdural space.

Question 3

E *Extradural haemorrhage (EDH)*
A hyperdense, biconvex, extra-axial (i.e outside the cerebral hemisphere) collection, overlying the occipital region is seen, compressing and displacing

the underlying brain. Haemorrhage occurs at the site of trauma, with laceration of a vessel (usually middle meningeal artery) and collection of blood within the extradural space.

A hypodense swirling pattern ('swirl sign') indicates active bleeding. EDH may cross the midline and dural attachments but rarely crosses sutures. Look for secondary effects such as herniation, contrecoup, SDH and contusions.

The patient needs urgent referral to the neurosurgeons for decompression. The classical clinical picture is of a patient suffering a head injury (often young healthy people), followed by a lucid interval and subsequent clinical and neurological deterioration.

Question 4

A *Intracerebral haemorrhage (ICH)*
The scan shows hypodensity mass centred on the right frontal lobe with surrounding low density (oedema). There is associated mass effect, with compression of the ipsilateral lateral ventricle.

Causes of ICH in the elderly include hypertension (often in basal ganglia), amyloid (often lobar bleed) and coagulopathy. Underlying conditions such as aneurysms, arteriovenous malformations (AVM) and tumours should also be considered, particularly in younger patients.

It is important not only to identify the ICH but also to look for causes (e.g. fractures, AVMs may be present) and consequences of the ICH (e.g. mass effect, hydrocephalus, brain herniation).

Question 5

B *Infarction*
The scan shows a hypodensity involving the grey and white matter in a left middle cerebral artery (MCA) and anterior cerebral artery (ACA) distribution. There is associated mass effect with compression of the ipsilateral lateral ventricle and midline shift to the right.

Early changes of a cerebrovascular accident (CVA) include loss of the grey-white matter differentiation. This is followed by gyral swelling, sulcal effacement, cytotoxic oedema with low attenuation seen on CT in the affected area. A hyperdense MCA is sometimes seen ('dense MCA sign') in MCA territory infarction. Haemorrhagic transformation can occur 2–3 days later with areas of high attenuation seen within the infarcted region. Over time the infarcted area becomes malacic and of very low density.

Question 6

C Pneumothorax

The lung edge is visible as a thin white line, with lucency outside it representing air in the pleural space. No lung markings are seen beyond the lung edge. A pneumothorax can occur spontaneously (classically in young, tall, thin men), following trauma and due to other rare causes. Look for mediastinal shift away from the affected side, representing a tension pneumothorax, which is a medical emergency requiring urgent decompression. In an ideal world, these should be picked up on clinical examination and treated prior to performing a chest X-ray.

Question 7

B Laparotomy

Air is seen below both hemidiaphragms consistent with pneumoperitoneum. This is a medical emergency and the patient needs an urgent surgical review. The definitive management is laparotomy. All other options would be helpful and an adjunct to definitive management.

A pneumoperitoneum represents gas within the peritoneal cavity resulting from a perforated viscus. Perforation of a duodenal/gastric ulcer, perforated appendix and trauma are possible causes.

This should not be confused with Chiladiti's syndrome where loops of bowel are interposed between liver and diaphragm, simulating a perforation.

Question 8

D Left lower lobe collapse

A triangular, retrocardiac opacity (representing the collapsed lower lobe) is seen which blurs the left hemidiaphragm. Signs to look for include other indications of volume loss, such as mediastinal shift to the left and a raised left hemidiaphragm. There may be slight lucency over the mid- to upper zones and a mild increase in rib spacing due to compensatory hyperexpansion of the left upper lobe.

Also look for causes of collapse which could be due to an obstructing hilar tumour. Mucous plugging and impacted foreign bodies can also cause collapse.

The left lower lobe collapses posteromedially, behind the heart. Blurring of the hemidiaphragm on the chest X-ray is due to the collapsed lower lobe abutting the hemidiaphragm. When two objects of similar density abut each other, the border between them is not seen; the margins can be identified when there is a difference in density. Hence, in normality the hemidiaphragm is visible as air (within aerated lung) abuts the hemidiaphragm. With collapse of the lung the air–diaphragm interface is lost, causing blurring of the hemidiaphragm. This is known as the silhouette sign.

Question 9

E *Left upper lobe collapse*

The radiograph shows a 'veil like' hazy opacification of the left hemithorax with upward migration of the left hilum. Other signs include para-aortic radiolucency in the left upper zone resulting from upward migration of the left lower lobe ('luftsichel sign').

As with any lobar collapse, look for causes such as an obstructing tumour. The patient will require a CT or bronchoscopy for further evaluation.

Question 10

D *Right upper lobe collapse*

The radiograph shows an obvious dense opacification of the right upper zone with a well-defined inferior border that has a 'reverse S shaped' configuration (Golden's S sign) signifying collapse of the right upper lobe secondary to an obstructing tumour.

Question 11

A *Right middle lobe collapse*

The radiograph shows an opacification in the right mid-zone, with blurring of the right heart border. The horizontal fissure is pulled down. This illustrates the 'silhouette sign': when two areas of similar radiodensity are touching, the interface is not visible. Thus, collapse or consolidation of the right middle lobe (which abuts the right heart border) will cause obscuration of the right heart border.

Pectus excavatum can cause a similar appearance on chest X-ray – look for sharp downward angulation of the anterior ribs.

Question 12

A *Diuretics*

There is bilateral perihilar air space opacification with small bilateral pleural effusions. Features are in keeping with pulmonary oedema.

Most patients with left ventricular failure have cardiomegaly. Early stages of fluid accumulation in the lung due to cardiogenic causes exhibit vascular redistribution, with the diameter of upper lobe veins being equal to or greater than that of the lower lobe veins (pulmonary venous hypertension). With increasing severity there is interstitial oedema as demonstrated by peribronch-ovascular cuffing, Kerley lines, unsharp central pulmonary vessels and effu-sions. Alveolar oedema with air space opacification occurs with further increase in pressures. The patient will require treatment with diuretics and nitrates.

Question 13

C Right pleural effusion

Homogenous opacification of the right lower zone, with a well-defined superior border and a meniscoid lateral edge. This represents fluid collected in the pleural space (between the parietal and visceral pleura). Possible causes include malignancy, infection, pulmonary oedema and trauma.

Other radiographic signs to look for include a hydropneumothorax (fluid and air in the pleural space demonstrated by a straight air–fluid level within the pneumothorax), a subpulmonic effusion (an apparently raised hemidiaph-ragm with the contour elevated laterally).

Depending on the clinical picture, the patient will often require aspiration of pleural fluid which is then analysed to look for a cause of the effusion. With a large effusion, the patient may require a chest drain to remove the fluid.

Question 14

B Antibiotics

The radiograph shows patchy, 'fluffy' opacification the right upper zone. Air bronchograms are seen within the opacification.

The radiographic appearance of consolidation is a result of material accumulating within the air spaces/alveoli. This could be pus due to infection, blood or fluid as result of pulmonary oedema or sometimes tumour. History and ancillary radiographic signs will establish the cause.

In the clinical context there is clinical and radiological suspicion of sepsis, so these changes represent pneumonia.

Question 15

A Left apical mass

There is a well-defined, round opacity in the left apex (see X-ray). There are many causes for lung nodules. Benign tumours (may have calcium or fat within them), infections (e.g. hydatid cysts), arteriovenous malformations (AVMs) and granulomas (usually smaller and multiple) are possibilities, but in an elderly smoker, bronchogenic carcinoma is the main concern. Metastases are a possibility but these are often multiple.

The patient needs further investigation with a staging CT for further assessment.

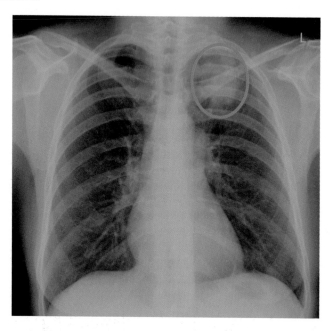

Question 16

C Cardiac arrhythmia

This patient has a dual chamber pacemaker. The pacemaker lies just under the skin and two leads pass (via the subclavian vein) to the right atrium and right ventricle where they attach via electrodes. The pacemaker provides electrical stimuli to enable contraction of the heart at the required rate.

Look for complications of pacemaker insertion such as a pneumothorax, fractures of the leads or pacemaker and other signs of cardiovascular disease.

Question 17

C Swallowed foreign body

There is a round, well-defined, highly radiodense object seen projected over the neck, in keeping with an ingested foreign body such as a coin. In view of stridor, the boy will need urgent assessment by the ENT surgical team. Surprisingly, these are sometimes very easy to overlook as they can be mistaken for metallic objects on the patient's body!

Question 18

D Anticoagulation

There is a filling defect in the main pulmonary artery extending into both the left and right pulmonary arteries, in keeping with pulmonary emboli (see arrow on figure, below).

Identify and follow the pulmonary arteries to look for filling defects caused by emboli. Other findings could include pulmonary infarction, consolidation and effusions. The patient requires assessment by the physicians with a view to anticoagulation.

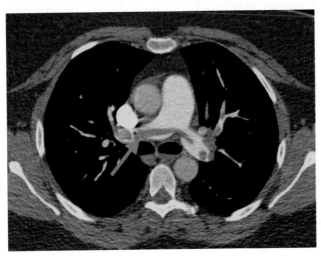

Question 19

B Small bowel obstruction

The abdominal X-ray shows central loops of dilated bowel with paucity of air in the distal bowel and no air in the rectum. Features are diagnostic of a small bowel obstruction (SBO). Note the presence of the valvulae conniventes (circled on X-ray), which encircle the small bowel – this features helps differentiate SBO from large bowel obstruction.

It would be useful to try and identify a 'cut-off' point where there is a transition from proximal dilated bowel to distal collapsed bowel, but this is often not possible on a plain radiograph. Causes of SBO include herniae and volvulus. In the current era, a CT would subsequently be performed for more detailed information.

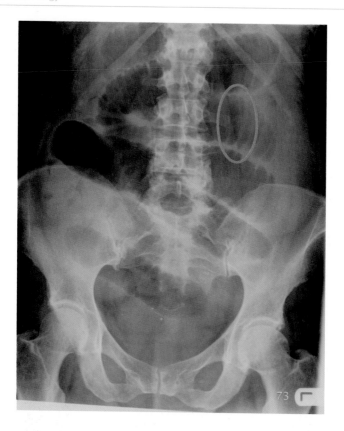

Question 20

C Pneumoperitoneum

Gas is seen on both sides of the bowel wall (Rigler's sign), in keeping with a perforated viscus. Other places to look for free air on an abdominal X-ray include around the falciform ligament, and the subhepatic and subdiaphragmatic regions. Unusual gas collections (particularly triangular-shaped areas of air) should raise a suspicion of pneumoperitoneum.

This patient may well be peritonitic and requires an urgent surgical review.

Question 21

C Large bowel obstruction

There are dilated loops of large bowel extending down to the distal sigmoid. Gas is not seen in the rectum. Only the colon is involved, suggesting that this is mechanical obstruction with a competent ileo-caecal valve.

Look for a 'cut-off point' that will demonstrate the point of obstruction (often not identified on plain radiography). The patient should remain nil by mouth and have a NG tube and IV fluids awaiting a surgical review. A toxic megacolon (colon >10 cm) requires urgent surgical review.

Note the lack of valvulae conniventes in the large bowel but the presence of haustral folds that shape the walls of the large bowel (circled on X-ray, below). Compare this radiograph with the one in Question 19 and familiarise yourself with the differences between large and small bowel obstruction.

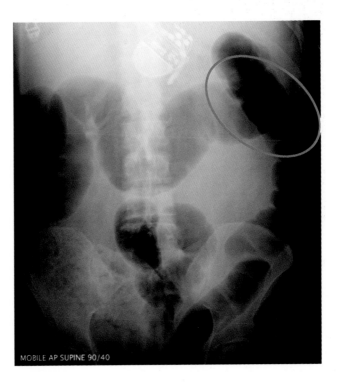

MOBILE AP SUPINE 90/40

Question 22

D Renal calculi

There are small, irregular, well-defined opacities seen overlying both kidneys (see arrows on X-ray). The right renal calculus is at the site of the pelvi-ureteric junction and is notorious in causing hydronephrosis. Ninety per cent of renal calculi are visible on plain radiographs. An IV urogram

(IVU) or ultrasound scan can demonstrate evidence of obstruction with hydronephrosis. The patient will need analgesia and a urological referral.

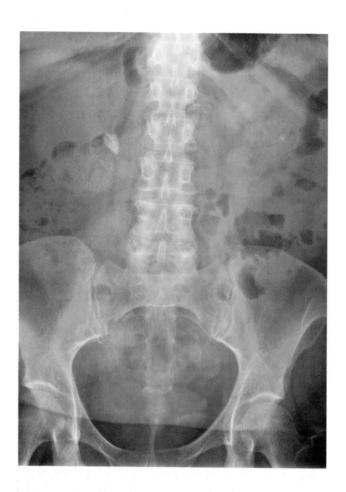

Question 23

E *Gallstones*

Well-defined calcific densities are projected over the right upper quadrant consistent with gallstones (see circle on X-ray). Around 10% of gallstones are visible on plain radiography. Abdominal X-ray is not the investigation of choice for cholelithiasis, but they are sometimes found incidentally on abdominal X-ray. Ultrasonography is the initial investigation for suspected gallstones.

A positive Murphy's sign can be seen in acute cholecystitis. This is performed by firmly placing a hand at the costal margin over the gallbladder and asking the patient to inspire deeply. If the gallbladder is inflamed, the patient will experience pain as the gallbladder descends and contacts the palpating hand. The same manoeuvre on the left upper quadrant should elicit no discomfort. This can be performed both at the bedside and in the radiology department using the ultrasound probe.

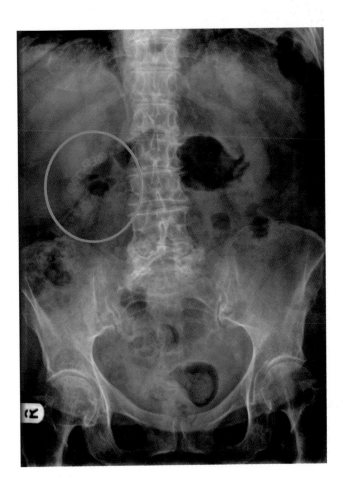

Question 24

C Refer him to the surgical team

The CT image shows a large abdominal aortic aneurysm. There are no obvious signs of rupture, however the clinical presentation is suggestive of impending rupture. Tachycardia and increasing pain are worrying and the patient should be referred to the surgical team for further assessment and possible surgery. Spontaneous rupture of an abdominal aortic aneurysm represents a true surgical emergency and is associated with a high mortality. Screening programmes for this condition using ultrasound scans have been established nationally.

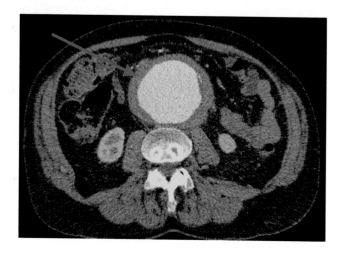

Question 25

A Diverticular disease

The barium enema image shows moderate diverticular disease involving the transverse and the descending colon. Diverticulae are seen as outpouchings from the colonic wall with some of them filling with contrast while others are filled with air. There is no stricture, benign or malignant, and there is no bowel wall thickening to suggest colitis.

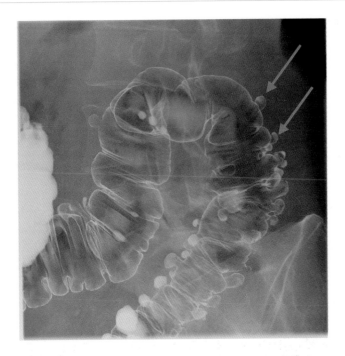

Question 26

E Malignant colorectal disease

The barium enema image shows the classical 'apple core' stricture of the recto-sigmoid in keeping with a malignant stricture. No diverticulae are seen in the image. In benign stricture, there will be smooth tapering of the colon rather than the irregular margins seen in this case.

6 General Surgery and Gastroenterology

Questions

Parveen Jayia, Petrut Gogalniceanu and Paraskevas A. Paraskeva

Question 1

A 52-year-old woman has been seen in A&E with recurrent episodes of right upper quadrant (RUQ) pain. She also complained of nausea and itching. On examination she is apyrexial, with guarding in the epigastrium area and RUQ but with no rebound tenderness. As part of her work-up, her liver function tests show:

Alkaline phosphatase (ALP) – 430 IU/L

Alanine aminotransferase (ALT) – 354 IU/L

Bilirubin – 34 μmol/L

Gamma-glutamyl transpeptidase (GGT) – 231 IU/L

International normalised ratio (INR) – 1.2

Albumin – 21 g/L

Amylase – 142 IU/L

1. What is the most likely diagnosis?
A. Hepatitis B
B. Obstructive jaundice
C. Hepatic failure
D. Ascending cholangitis
E. Acute pancreatitis

2. What is the most appropriate next step in her management?
A. Keep nil by mouth (NBM)
B. CT angiogram (not helical CT)
C. Endoscopic retrograde cholangiopancreatography (ERCP)
D. Ultrasound (US) of the abdomen
E. Abdominal radiograph

Clinical Data Interpretation for Medical Finals: Single Best Answer Questions, First Edition.
Edited by Philip Socrates Pastides and Parveen Jayia.
© 2012 Philip Socrates Pastides and Parveen Jayia. Published 2012 by John Wiley & Sons, Ltd.

Question 2

A 45-year-old smoker who is well known to the department is admitted with sudden-onset epigastric pain with nausea and vomiting. On examination he is pyrexial, tender over the epigastrium. The abdominal radiograph shows a loop of dilated small bowel. Erect chest radiograph shows basal atelactasis. His blood results are as follows:

White cell count (WCC) – 15.4 × 10⁹/L	ALP – 43 IU/L
Haemoglobin (Hb) – 11.2 g/dL	ALT – 14 IU/L
Platelets – 354 × 10⁹/L	Albumin – 15 g/L
Creatinine – 112 mmol/L	Corrected calcium – 1.19 mmol/L
Urea – 18 mmol/L	Amylase – 1223 u/L

1. What is the most likely diagnosis?

A. Acute cholestasis
B. Biliary colic
C. Chronic pancreatitis
D. Perforated peptic ulcer
E. Acute pancreatitis

The patient's condition begins to deteriorate [blood pressure (BP) 86/74 mmHg, heart rate (HR) 112/min, respiration rate (RR) 28/min] whilst in A&E. The surgical SHO continues with fluid resuscitation, and an arterial blood gas is performed, with results as follows:

pH – 7.31
PCO_2 – 3.8 kPa
PO2 – 7.9 kPa
Lactate – 4.2 mmol/L
Base excess (BE) – –3.9 mmol/L
HCO_3 – 19.2

2. What is the next appropriate step?

A. Immediate laparotomy
B. Urgent CT scan
C. Oxygen therapy, fluid resuscitation and intensive care (ITU) referral
D. ERCP
E. Magnetic resonance cholangiopancreatography (MRCP)

Question 3

A 22-year-old man presents to clinic with fatigue and abdominal pain. He informs you that he has had an increased frequency of bowel movement over the past 3 months with loose stool that is sometimes mixed with blood and mucus. He is extremely anxious that this is affecting his studies. On examination he has mild generalised tenderness. His GP has completed the following investigations:

Hb – 9.8 g/dL   Bilirubin – 15 μmol/L
WCC – 16.8 × 10⁹/L   Albumin – 18 g/L
Platelets – 253 × 10⁹/L   Amylase 41 IU/L
Creatinine – 78 mmol/L   Urea – 4.2 mmol/L
ALT – 17 IU/L   C-reactive protein (CRP) – 172 mg/L
ALP – 32 IU/L

His abdominal X-ray (post-barium follow-through) is shown below:

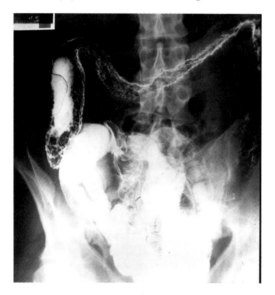

1. What is the likely diagnosis?

A. Diverticular disease
B. Whipple's disease
C. Crohn's disease
D. Ulcerative colitis
E. Infective diarrhoea

2. Which investigation can confirm the diagnosis and differentiate between different types of the disease?

A. CT scan abdomen/pelvis
B. Barium enema
C. Colonoscopy
D. Flexible sigmoidoscopy
E. Stool cultures

Question 4

You are asked by A&E to review a 43-year-old woman who underwent a laparoscopic cholecystectomy 6 weeks ago. She has now presented with increasing epigastric pain. She has also noticed that her urine is dark and her stools have become pale. She is complaining of nausea without vomiting and has opened her bowels once this morning. Her PMH is unremarkable. On examination she is noted to be jaundiced and is tender over the RUQ and epigastric area. Her scar is healing well. Her investigations are as follows:

HB – 16.3 g/dL
WCCC – 8.2 × 10^9/L
Platelets – 189 × 10^9/L
Creatinine – 76 mmol/L
ALT – 159 IU/L
ALP – 455 IU/L

Bilirubin – 108 µmol/L
Albumin – 35 g/L
Amylase – 68 IU/L
Urea – 2.5 mmol/L
CRP – 22 mg/L

1. What is the most likely cause of the patient's pain?

A. Chronic pancreatitis
B. Common bile duct stone
C. Biliary stricture
D. Ascending cholangitis
E. Primary sclerosing cholangitis

2. What is the next most appropriate test?

A. MRCP followed by ERCP
B. ERCP
C. US
D. CT scan abdomen and pelvis
E. Serial observations and examination

Question 5

A 72-year-old man, known to be hypertensive and a heavy smoker, presents to A&E with left loin pain radiating to the groin. He informs you that it has been present for 2 days and is no longer managed with analgesia and is constantly present. Urine analysis shows haematuria. On examination you note he has cool peripherally and abdominal examination shows tenderness centrally. His observations are as follows:

Temperature – 37.6 °C
HR – 110/min
BP – 106/78 mmHg
Sats – 91% on room air

1. What is the likely diagnosis?
A. Renal colic
B. Pyelonephritis
C. Diverticulitis
D. Acute pancreatitis
E. Abdominal aortic aneurysm (AAA)

The following CT scan of the abdomen is obtained urgently, after the patient was optimised:

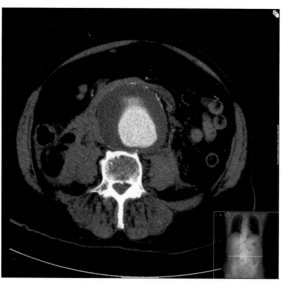

2. What is the diagnosis?

A. Renal calculi

B. Perinephric inflammation due to urinary tract infection (UTI)

C. Ruptured abdominal aortic aneurysm

D. Small bowel obstruction

E. Diverticular disease

Question 6

A 45-year-old obese woman with a strong alcohol history presents to A&E with colicky abdominal pain not relieved by paracetamol. Direct questioning reveals that she has had similar episodes of pain in the last 4 weeks. She denies any fevers, but on examination you feel a mass in her right hypochondrium that is mildly tender. An urgent US of her abdomen is arranged. Her blood profile is now available as follows:

ALT – 89 IU/L

Bilirubin – 32 μmol/L

Amylase – 62 IU/L

ALP – 155 IU/L

HB – 10.2 g/dL

WCC – 5.6 × 10^9/L

Platelets – 321 × 10^9/L

What is the most likely cause of this presentation?

A. Acute cholecystitis

B. Choledocholithiasis

C. Mucocele of gallbladder

D. Peptic ulcer disease

E. Acute pancreatitis

Question 7

An 82-year-old man is admitted to A&E from the local residential care home with colicky generalised abdominal pain. He is incontinent of urine and the healthcare staff notice that his stools have been looser and that there is some blood mixed with it. He has a long-standing history of constipation and use of laxatives. On examination there is marked abdominal distension, diffuse tenderness and high-pitched bowel sounds. An abdominal radiograph is performed and is shown below:

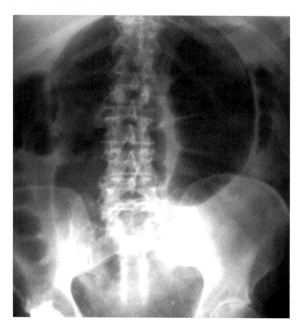

What is the diagnosis?
A. Small bowel obstruction
B. Toxic megacolon
C. Sigmoid volvulus
D. Abdominal aortic aneurysm
E. Distended bladder

Question 8

You are asked to see a 78-year-old woman admitted to the care of the elderly ward with a history of recurrent falls. Looking through her admission notes you establish this is her third admission in the last month. On this admission to A&E she was noted to be tachycardic and hypotensive. The referring doctor informs you that she is still complaining of right-sided abdominal pain and has been noted to have had some dark red per rectal bleeding mixed with stool. She is also known to have a loud ejection systolic murmur on cardiac auscultation. Endoscopic investigations have been performed. Her investigations are as follows:

Upper GI endoscopy – mild duodenitis

Colonoscopy – small flat red lesions in caecum and ascending colon

Hb – 6.7 g/dL

Mean cell volume (MCV) – 75 fL

Mean cell haemoglobin (MCH) – 85 g/dL

WCC – 4.5×10^9/L

Platelets – 425×10^9/L

Urea – 4.3 mmol/L

Creatinine – 91 mmol/L

Albumin – 24 g/L

ALP – 32 IU/L

ALT – 15 IU/L

What is the most likely cause of her anaemia?

A. Diverticulitis
B. Colonic carcinoma
C. Anal fissure
D. Angiodysplasia
E. Diverticular disease

Question 9

The A&E registrar asks you to see a 25-year-old man who has presented with lower abdominal pain, distension and vomiting. He has not opened his bowels for 2 days. Review of his notes shows a recent admission with right iliac fossa pain and treatment with antibiotics. His investigations and abdominal X-ray are shown:

US abdomen – difficult scan due to overlying loops of small bowel

Hb – 9.2 g/dL

White cell count – 11.4×10^9/L

Urea – 8.5 mmol/L

Creatinine – 113 mmol/L

C-reactive protein – 56

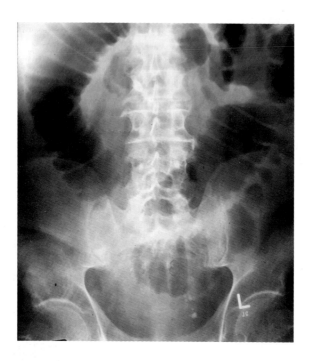

What is the most likely cause of his symptoms?
A. Peptic ulcer disease
B. Urinary tract infection
C. Appendicitis
D. Intussusception
E. Diverticular disease

Question 10

A 35-year-old male tennis player with a history of chronic knee pain presents with severe upper abdominal pain associated with vomiting. On examination his abdomen is rigid and bowel sounds are absent. His observations are recorded below:
Temperature – 37.7 °C
RR – 28/min
Saturations – 92% on room air
HR – 115 beats/min

BP – 95/60 mmHg

The erect chest X-ray and abdominal X-rays are shown below:

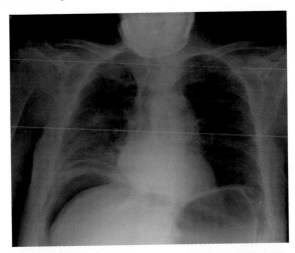

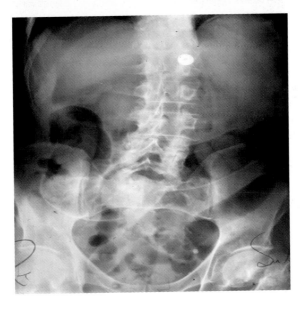

What is the most likely cause of his abdominal pain?
A. Pancreatitis
B. Acute cholecystitis
C. Perforated peptic ulcer
D. Angiodysplasia
E. Small bowel obstruction

Question 11

A 52-year-old heavy smoker is referred to the clinic by his GP with a history of left-sided calf pain brought on by walking and relieved by rest. His walking distance has been reduced to 250 yards over the course of the past 4 months.

In clinic you perform an ankle-brachial pressure index (ABPI) and obtain a result of 0.7. You notice that his left leg is warm but you are not able to palpate his foot pulses.

What is the next best step in his management?
A. Admit for analgesia and further investigations
B. Recommend an outpatient duplex study and see again in clinic
C. Recommend outpatient duplex & angiogram and see again in clinic
D. Request an outpatient CT scan of the lower limbs and see again in clinic
E. Give lifestyle advice (smoking cessation, healthy diet), increase exercise, commence aspirin and see in clinic.

Question 12

A patient suffering from diabetes develops rest pain at night in his left foot. He undergoes a digital subtraction angiogram of his affected limb. Below is one image from this investigation:

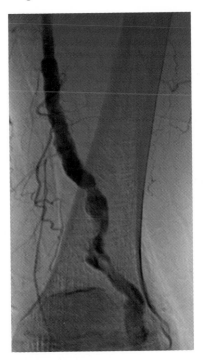

What does the image show?

A. Occlusion of the external iliac artery
B. Stenosis of the internal iliac artery
C. Stenosis in the common femoral artery
D. Stenosis of the superficial femoral artery (SFA) and popliteal artery
E. Aneurysm with thrombosis in the popliteal artery

Question 13

A 67-year-old woman is rushed into A&E by her worried family with agonising diffuse abdominal pain. She suffered a similar episode after food a day ago, but is complaining that this pain is worse. She is known to suffer from ischaemic heart disease and hypertension. She takes anti-hypertensive medication along with aspirin. On examination she is cool peripherally, has an irregular heart rhythm, is diffusely tender on mild abdominal palpation and has absent bowel sounds. Her pain appears inconsistent with findings on abdominal palpation.

Her blood profile is shown below:

WCC 12.3 × 10^9/L

Hb 9.2 g/dL

Platelets 376 × 10^9/L

Urea 10.8 mmol/L

Creatinine 172 mmol/L

Albumin 31 g/L

ALT 54 IU/L

ALP 101 IU/L

Bilirubin 20 μmol/L

CRP 35 mg/L

Her arterial blood gas is as follows:

pH – 7.31

PCO_2 – 4.1 kPa

PO_2 – 10.2 (on room air) kPa

HCO_3 – 21 mEq/L

BE – -4.1 mmol/L

Lactate – 5.2 mmol/L

Her ECG shows fast atrial fibrillation (AF).

What is the most likely cause of her pain?

A. Bowel obstruction

B. Perforated peptic ulcer

C. Aortic aneurysm rupture

D. Mesenteric ischaemia/ischaemic bowel

E. Inflammatory bowel disease

Question 14

A 23-year-old man presents to his GP with a 4-day history of right-sided groin pain radiating to his testis associated with dysuria, frequency and fevers. He denies any urethral discharge but is sexually active. On examination he has noticeable testicular tenderness. His abdominal examination is negative. His urine analysis is as follows:

Leukocytes 3 +

Nitrates 3 +

Blood 2 +

The GP is worried and sends the patient to be seen by the surgical registrar on call. His blood results are below:

WBC – 15.3 × 10^9/L

Hb – 13.2 g/dL

Platelets – 213 × 10^9/L

CRP – 62 mg/L

On examination, you note that his testis is soft but mildly swollen with some scrotal erythema. There is extreme tenderness on the posterior aspect of his right testicle. The surgical registrar orders an US of his testis, the report of which is as follows:

US report – increased Doppler wave pulsation is noted in the right testis; small amount of free fluid is seen around the testis.

What is the most likely cause?
A. Testicular torsion
B. Epididymitis
C. Urinary tract infection
D. Orchitis
E. Epididymal-orchitis

Question 15

A 20-year-old college students presents with a week-long history of head-ache, malaise and a recently noticed swelling in the neck that is more painful on eating. His also anxious about his right-sided testicular pain. On exami-nation he is tender over the right angle of his mandible. He has a maculo-papular rash and has a tender smooth right testicle. His observations are as follows:
Temperature – 37.7 °C
HR – 96 beats/min
RR – 18/min
BP – 118/86 mmHg
Urine analysis – leucocytes 1 +, nitrates negative, blood negative

What is the most likely cause of his pain?
A. Testicular torsion
B. Orchitis
C. Urinary tract infection
D. Mastoiditis
E. Mumps

Question 16

A 48-year-old woman presents with a 2-month history of RUQ pain increasing in frequency and severity over the past 24 hours. She complains of feeling 'hot and cold' and has had some weight loss of late. She has a previous history of gallstone disease. On examination she has yellow sclera and is tender over her RUQ with mild rebound. Her observations are as follows:

Temperature – 38.2 °C
HR – 105 beats/min
BP –119/76 mmHg
Her blood results are as follows:

WCC – 14.6 × 10⁹/L

Neutrophils – 12.3 × 10⁹/L

Hb – 12.5 g/dL

Platelets – 301 × 10⁹/L

ALT – 298 IU/L

ALP – 214 IU/L

Bilirubin – 47 μmol/L

Albumin – 25 g/L

Amylase – 145 IU/L

Urea – 9.2 mmol/L

Creatinine – 110 mmol/L

What is the likely diagnosis in this patient?

A. Retained common bile duct stone
B. Autoimmune hepatitis
C. Postoperative bile leak
D. Ascending cholangitis
E. Cholangiocarcinoma

General Surgery and Gastroenterology

Answers

Question 1

1. B *Obstructive jaundice*

Definitions:

- Cholelithiasis – stone formation in the gallbladder
- Choledocholithiasis – the presence of gallstones in the common bile duct
- Cholestasis – failure of bile flow; the obstruction to bile flow can be either intrahepatic or extra-hepatic.
- Cholecystitis – inflammation of the gallbladder
- Cholangitis – inflammation of the biliary tree

In intrahepatic cholestasis there is a failure in one of the three steps in bilirubin metabolism (uptake, conjugation or excretion). Disease such as viral hepatitis or drug-induced hepatitis, biliary cirrhosis or alcoholic liver disease should be considered.

Extrahepatic obstruction can occur within the ducts or come about as a result of external compression. The commonest cause is gallstones, but others, such as inflammation, malignancy or strictures within the ducts, need to be considered. Females are most likely to be affected by gallstones (approximately 50% by age 75 years) mostly due to oestrogen which, forms bile from cholesterol.

In obstructive jaundice, bilirubin is always elevated. ALP (a membrane-bound enzyme) found in the bile canaliculi can be increased to three to five times the upper limit in extrahepatic obstruction. ALT is predominantly found in the liver hepatocytes and elevations are associated with hepatocyte damage secondary to intrahepatic obstruction of bile flow or liver injury.

As a rule of thumb:

- In hepatic jaundice or liver disease ALT > ALP, with a high bilirubin (e.g. viral hepatitis)
- In post-hepatic jaundice ALP > ALT, with a high bilirubin (e.g. obstructive jaundice secondary to liver disease).

2. D *US of the abdomen*

Plain radiographs are limited in detecting abnormalities in the biliary system as calculi are not visualised because few are radio-opaque. CT is usually more accurate as it can inform the clinician as to exact cause and the level of obstruction. However, it exposes the patient to radiation and cannot visualise the common bile duct (CBD) as well as can US.

Ultrasound is associated with 95% sensitivities in visualising the biliary system; it is regarded as the modality of choice. ERCP is used for both diagnostic and therapeutic purposes as it combines both endoscopic and radiological modalities. It is associated with complications such as pancreatitis, reactions to contrast material, perforation and sepsis and therefore it is always better to assess the patient initially with a non-invasive modality such as US.

Question 2

1. E *Acute pancreatitis*

The patient is well known to A&E, as many patients who have a long-standing problem with alcohol usually are. Acute pancreatitis occurs when there is an imbalance in cellular homeostasis when there is damage to the acinar cell. The leading cause in the UK is gallstones (40%) and alcohol (c. 35%). The other causes can be remembered by mnemonic GETSMASHED:

- Gallstones
- Ethanol
- Trauma (abdominal)
- Steroids
- Mumps (Epstein–Barr, measles)
- Autoimmune (systemic lupus erythematosus)
- Scorpion bites
- Hypercalcaemia/hyperlipidaemia/hypertriglyceridaemia/hypothermia
- ERCP
- Drugs [non-steroidal anti-inflammatory drugs (NSAIDs), diuretics, azathioprine].

Serum amylase (and lipase) is usually increased more than threefold. However, amylase is not specific to pancreatitis and can also be increased in other abdominal pathologies such as small bowel obstruction, mesenteric ischaemia, perforated gastric ulcer, renal failure and even ectopic pregnancies. In this case there is little derangement in liver function tests, suggesting that this pancreatitis is unlikely to be due to gallstones, and more likely to do with alcohol. Abdominal radiographs are useful to exclude other pathologies such as perforated viscus and in some cases the inflammation around the pancreas can cause a localised ileus, giving rise to a sentinel loop of small bowel as seen on the abdominal X-ray.

2. C *Oxygen therapy, fluid resuscitation and intensive care (ITU) referral*
In patients with pancreatitis and organ failure the mortality rate can be as high as 30–40%. Despite patients being admitted under the care of surgeons, the management is medical, with the focus on organ support, fluid hydration, electrolyte replacement and appropriate monitoring. The latter may only be appropriate in an ITU setting. The patients should receive cross-sectional imaging (CT) 3–4 days after the onset of pancreatitis in order to rule out pancreatic ischaemia or the formation of abscesses if no clear improvement is seen. In the case of this patient with metabolic acidosis, option C is the sensible option.

Question 3

1. C *Crohn's disease*
There is a bimodal distribution to Crohn's disease with the first peak occurring at 15–30 years of age and the second occurring after 60 years. The majority of patients will be diagnosed in the first peak with males twice as likely to be affected. Patients will present with low-grade pyrexia, abdominal pain and generalised weakness. The abdominal pain will be right-sided if the terminal ileum is affected. If the colon is involved, there may be stool mixed with blood and mucus (the latter being more likely in ulcerative colitis). Blood results can show anaemia and leucocytosis and raised CRP in response to inflammation, malabsorption or even in presence of abscess formation. Radiological imaging (in the form of barium or gastrograffin contrast enemas) is useful in assessing the severity and in determining the location of disease. Small bowel studies may show strictures, deep penetrating ulceration (rose thorn ulcers) and cobblestone mucosal surfaces (skip lesions – areas of healthy mucosa next to diseased bowel).

2. C *Colonoscopy*
Diagnosis requires histological evidence of inflammatory bowel disease through endoscopic biopsies. The only investigation that will assist in this is a full colonoscopy. CT scan is useful to assess the extent of fistulae and abscesses. Stool cultures are needed to exclude infectious aetiologies such as *Clostridium difficile*. Non-caseating granulomas with transmural involvement (full thickness) are diagnostic histological findings. Barium enemas (to assess

colonic involvement) should ideally never be performed in an acute episode of inflammatory bowel disease.

Question 4

1. B *Common bile duct stone*

The patient has presented with symptoms that are suggestive of obstructive jaundice, as indicated by her elevated liver function tests and her pale stools and dark urine. The complications of laparoscopic cholecystectomy include damage to the common bile duct resulting in biliary leak or bile duct stricture formation. The former would result in the patient being systemically unwell with a leucocytosis; patients also usually experience pyrexia. The latter can occur in 0.1–1% of cholecystectomies and therefore is considered uncommon. In the majority of these patients, it is important to exclude retained gallstones in the CBD.

2. C *US*

Initial assessment of retained CBD stones requires imaging of the CBD to identify any dilatation using US. This can be followed by an ERCP if there is evidence of obstruction or by an MRCP if the diagnosis is not clear. US is a non-invasive test that is used to assess the pancreas, liver and biliary tract. The common bile duct should be approximately 4 mm in diameter and, in obstruction, can increase to 12–14 mm.

Question 5

1. E *AAA*

Abdominal aortic aneurysm is a disease that typically affects men with a history of hypertension and smoking. Whilst a number of risk factors have been suggested, over 90% of AAAs are thought to be the result of a degenerative process that commences due to atherosclerosis, affecting the medium and large blood vessels. Other causes include infections (mycotic aneurysms) and connective tissue disorders (Marfan's disease). Most patients will be asymptomatic but patients with rupture can present with a range of symptoms such as back pain, loin pain, groin pain or even collapse. In this patient he is hypotensive and tachycardic and has pain that is progressively getting worse. These symptoms should always raise suspicion.

2. C *Ruptured abdominal aortic aneurysm*

This is an infrarenal aneurysm. Note the obvious contrast (bright white area) within the aorta surrounded by haematoma (grey area).

Question 6

C Mucocele of gallbladder

A mucocele of a gallbladder develops from an outlet obstruction, commonly due to a stone in the cystic duct or gallbladder neck. A chronic obstruction results in distension of the gallbladder and will typically contain either clear watery liquid or mucoid secretions (mucocele) instead of bile, as the bile pigment is usually reabsorbed. With recurrent attacks of cholecystitis there may be wall thickening. The patient will present with RUQ pain, nausea and vomiting, and on examination there is a palpable tender mass. If the patient is febrile, acute cholecystitis or empyema of the gallbladder should be excluded.

Rules of thumb:

- Painful post-hepatic jaundice – biliary obstruction, most likely caused by gallstone disease
- Painless post-hepatic jaundice – biliary tree obstruction secondary to a neoplastic process (e.g. pancreatic head adenocarcinoma).

Remember Courvoisier's law which states that in the presence of jaundice and a non-tender distended gallbladder, the jaundice is unlikely to be caused by gallstone disease. This is because in gallstone disease the patient has recurrent episodes of cholecystitis which leads to thickening of gallbladder wall. Consequently any blockage of bile flow generating backpressure into the gallbladder will not be able to distend it. An acutely distended gallbladder suggests the presence of local neoplasm, such as adenocarcinoma of the pancreatic head to cholangiocarcinoma. Blockage in these circumstances in a previously non-inflamed gland leads to a distended and palpable structure.

Question 7

C Sigmoid volvulus

A volvulus occurs where there is an abnormal rotation in a loop of bowel around its mesenteric pedicle. This can lead to acute or subacute bowel obstruction, as well as infarction of a bowel segment should its blood supply be interrupted by the rotation of the mesentery. It will account for approximately 8–15% of all large bowel obstructions, with the sigmoid being the most common site. The transverse colon and caecum can also be affected, as they are not retroperitoneal structures. The most common cause of sigmoid volvulus is chronic constipation, which can cause the bowel loops to undergo progressive dilation and thus lengthening, allowing it to twist at the base of its mesentery. The patient will present with tender abdominal distension in the acute situation.

Question 8

D *Angiodysplasia*

Patients with angiodysplasia will present with active gastrointestinal bleeding in less than 10% of cases, with the majority being asymptomatic. It is a degenerative lesion of blood vessels commonly associated with ageing. Patients will often have chronic, low-grade bleeding, which will often spontaneously resolve but leave the patient haemodynamically compromised. In about 15% of cases, the patient will present with acute haemorrhage and will need urgent medical assessment. Some patients will also have diverticular disease. The immediate management for any bleeding patient is to ensure appropriate IV access, to assess the volume lost and to replace accordingly. In this case the blood profile shows she is anaemic. Once stable the patient will be investigated with a colonoscopy, which shows the characteristic picture of small flat red lesions usually affecting the right side of the colon.

Question 9

C *Appendicitis*

Acute appendicitis is the most common causes of an acute surgical abdomen. Approximately 50% of patients will present with classic signs of central abdominal pain radiating to the right iliac fossa, and the rest will present with an atypical history that makes it a diagnostic challenge. This is mostly determined by the location of the tip of the appendix, which can be retro-caecal, pelvic, pre-ileal and post-ileal. The most common complication of appendicitis is rupture, which may result in generalised peritonitis. In some cases, an appendicular mass (omentum surrounding the appendix) may form when the appendix becomes gangrenous. This is a protective mechanism to prevent generalised peritonitis if the appendix does rupture. In rare cases, peri-appendicular inflammation can cause adhesions, which can result in small bowel obstruction. The abdominal radiograph shows dilation of the small bowel and in this case it is secondary to appendicitis.

Question 10

C *Perforated peptic ulcer*

The patient with a history of chronic knee pain is most likely to be self-medicating with NSAIDs, such as ibuprofen. These are prostaglandin inhibitors. Endogenous prostaglandins protect the gastric mucosa and their inhibition increases the risk of gastritis and gastric ulceration. When a patient presents with rigidity, a perforated viscus must always be excluded. In such cases, an *erect* chest radiograph (after 30 min) and abdominal film should be taken. Pneumoperitoneum indicates rupture or perforation of a hollow viscus in up to 90% of cases. Other causes could be peritoneal dialysis, recent endoscopy or vigorous respiratory resuscitation. Rigler (an American radiologist) first described in 1941 that patients with extensive intraperitoneal air would have both sides of the bowel wall visible in an abdominal radiograph. Normally gas would only outline the luminal surface of the bowel wall and not the serosal side. This is called Rigler's sign.

Question 11

E Give lifestyle advice (smoking cessation, healthy diet), increase exercise, commence aspirin and see in clinic

This is a typical case of lower limb intermittent claudication due to peripheral arterial vascular disease. The presence of arterial stenosis will result in impaired blood flow to muscles during periods of exercise. Eventually the metabolic demands of the muscle exceed blood flow and symptoms of claudication result. Intermittent claudication pain should be reproducible, should be within the same location and should be eased by the same period of rest. It is most common in men, with smoking being the most significant risk factor (as seen in this case). Other risk factors include hypertension, diabetes mellitus, hypercholesterolaemia and family history of vascular disease. In the history it is important to exclude other diseases that present similarly such as:

- Osteoarthritis – variable pain pattern
- Spinal stenosis – usually bilateral, associated with numbness and tingling of the legs. Worsened by standing erect or walking downhill, and relieved by flexing or lying down
- Venous disease – usually described as a dull ache that occur after periods of standing erect; not known to be caused following exercise
- Deep venous thrombosis.

$$\text{Ankle-brachial pressure index(ABPI)} = \frac{\text{ankle systolic pressure}}{\text{brachial systolic pressure}}$$

An ABPI < 0.95 usually signifies peripheral arterial disease. Symptoms of claudication tend to occur in the range 0.5–0.9, whereas rest pain and critical ischaemia usually occur with an ABPI < 0.5. ABPI > 1.2/1.3 implies arterial calcification and can occur in diabetes.

Treatment initially involves reducing cardiovascular risk, improving exercise tolerance, commencing anti-platelet therapy (aspirin) and considering starting a statin. Other forms of imaging such as duplex ultrasound can be arranged as an outpatient to map the location and severity of vascular stenosis or occlusion

Question 12

D *Stenosis of the superficial femoral artery (SFA) and popliteal artery*

Angiography is performed to image the arterial tree and is usually performed when an intervention is planned. In this image there is stenosis in the left SFA and popliteal artery. This goes together with the history.

Question 13

D *Mesenteric ischaemia/ischaemic bowel*

Ischaemic bowel can present acutely with a sudden onset of diffuse abdominal pain that is poorly localised with a relatively normal abdominal examination. There may be absent bowel sounds (in the case of ileus and advancing ischaemia) and blood per rectum. Patients usually have a strong cardiac history (as in this case) and may have experienced intestinal angina (postprandial pain ~30 min afterwards). The most common cause is an acute embolic event from a proximal source. In this case we know the ECG shows atrial fibrillation, so the likeliest cause is a thrombus from the left heart. Valve disease (infective endocarditis) and ventricular or aortic aneurysms can also predispose to embolisation. In the chronic setting, patients will present with a prolonged history of postprandial pain and as a result have extreme weight loss and appear malnourished due to a fear of food. In these patients there may be a collateral blood flow to the bowel and they may not experience the same level of symptoms (not always the case). In these patients, faecal occult bleeding occurs due to sloughing of ischaemic bowel mucosa, resulting in ischaemic colitis.

In the acute setting the patient needs to be resuscitated aggressively and taken for emergency laparotomy for resection of the affected bowel segment. Surgical embolectomy may be performed. Postoperative identification of the embolus is required, using echocardiography. Mortality is usually greater than 60%. The high lactate in this case is indicative of an underlying metabolic ischaemic event.

Question 14

B *Epididymitis*

Epididymitis is an inflammation of the epididymis. This is a coiled vessel located in the posterior aspect of the testicle that connects the testicle to the vas deferens. Inflammation is usually due to an infection caused by *Escherichia coli*, or, in sexually active men, *Chlamydia trachomatis* and *Neisseria gonorrhoeae*. It usually affects males over the age of 19 and is caused by retrograde spread of the microorganisms. Patients will present with pain localised to the epididymis on examination, urinary frequency and fevers, and some may complain of urethral discharge. It is important to exclude testicular torsion first, as it can occur in this age group. Patients usually have a more acute history of pain (< 24 hours), may have a history of trauma and on examination may have an elevated oedematous testicle. The surgical registrar has ordered the US to exclude a torsion, which would show diminished/absent blood flow if there was a torsion. Treatment of epididymitis encompasses analgesia and antibiotics.

Question 15

E Mumps

This patient has experienced classic prodromal symptoms (headache, malaise) which can last for up 5–7 days before other symptoms appear. These symptoms depend on the organ affected but most commonly involve the following:

- Parotid gland is most commonly affected and can be uni/bilaterally involved. The patient may complain of tenderness over the jaw angle and experience pain after eating.
- Testicles – orchitis occurs in half of the male patients and is usually unilateral (30% bilateral).
- Central nervous system – results in meningitis (worryingly, half may be asymptomatic). Male adults seem to be at a higher risk of this.
- Rarely the joints can be affected and some patients may experience sudden hearing loss due to eighth nerve involvement. Female patients may complain of abdominal pain secondary to ovarian inflammation. The patient remains infectious for up to 4–5 days from the onset of parotitis. Treatment is supportive and the patient contacts should be counselled for vaccination.

Question 16

D Ascending cholangitis

Ascending cholangitis is a surgical emergency that is caused by a bacterial infection of the biliary tract resulting from biliary stasis. This is most commonly due to the presence of stones or recent biliary tract manipulation (ERCP) but can be due to strictures and pancreatitis. Most are due to aerobic

Gram-negative bacterial infections (*E. coli*, *Klebsiella*, *Pseudomonas*). Less than a third of patients will present with classic Charcot's triad:
- right upper quadrant pain
- clinical jaundice
- swinging pyrexia.

The majority of patients will have fever and jaundice. Older patients may present with non-specific confusion or malaise. Blood cultures should be sent for this patient as she is pyrexial and she should be kept nil by mouth, have IV fluids and broad-spectrum antibiotics. The blood profile shows an obstructive jaundice, most likely due to gallstones. The patient may need endoscopic biliary decompression with ERCP or operative bile duct exploration. Untreated cholangitis can be fatal.

7 Musculoskeletal Medicine and Trauma

Questions

Philip S. Pastides and Parminder Johal

Question 1

A 68-year-old woman fell onto her outstretched arm. The injury is closed and there is no neurovascular deficit (radiographs are shown below).

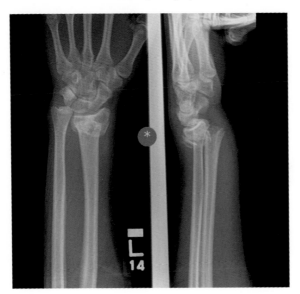

Clinical Data Interpretation for Medical Finals: Single Best Answer Questions, First Edition.
Edited by Philip Socrates Pastides and Parveen Jayia.
© 2012 Philip Socrates Pastides and Parveen Jayia. Published 2012 by John Wiley & Sons, Ltd.

Which one of the following features is not included in this injury?
A. Dinner fork deformity
B. Volar displacement of the distal radius
C. Radial tilt (loss of inclination)
D. Radial shortening
E. Comminution at the fracture site

Question 2

A 54-year-old woman fell of her bicycle and landed awkwardly onto her ankle. Her ankle looks clearly deformed. There is no skin damage or neurovascular deficit. Her radiograph is shown below:

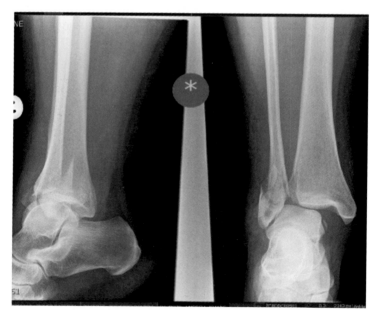

1. What does the radiograph show?
A. No fractures but subluxation of the ankle joint
B. Distal fibula fracture (Weber A) and subluxation of the ankle joint
C. Distal fibula fracture (Weber B) and subluxation of the ankle joint
D. Distal fibula fracture (Weber C) and subluxation of the ankle joint
E. Trimalleolar fracture

The patient is booked for theatre the following day.

2. What is the most appropriate treatment before the patient is taken to the ward and whilst awaiting the operation?

A. Immobilisation in the present position in a plaster back slab and elevation

B. Skeletal traction and elevation of the limb

C. Immobilisation in the present position in full plaster cast and elevation

D. Closed reduction and immobilise in plaster back slab and elevation

E. Measurement of compartment pressures in the limb until theatre

Question 3

A 67-year-old man has been complaining of worsening knee pain over the past few years. His pain is worse on the left side and has now started to wake him at night. His most recent radiographs are shown below:

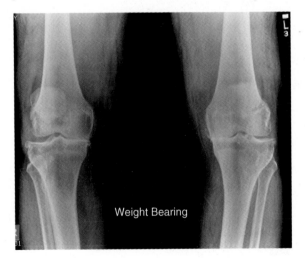

Weight Bearing

Which of the following is not specifically a radiological feature of osteoarthritis?

A. Loss of joint space

B. Osteophyte formation

C. Subchondral sclerosis

D. Varus deformity of the knee

E. Bony cyst formation

Question 4

An 81-year-old woman slips in her bedroom after getting up to go to the toilet at night. She falls onto her right side and is unable to weight bear. She has no other major medical co-morbidities. Her radiograph is shown below:

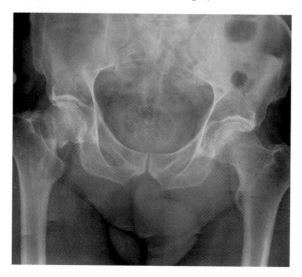

What is the most appropriate treatment for her injury?
A. Cannulated screws
B. Hemiarthroplasty of the right hip
C. Right total hip replacement
D. Conservative treatment with physiotherapy
E. Right dynamic hip screw

Question 5

A 76-year-old woman falls onto her hip whilst ice skating with her grand-children. She is unable to weight-bear on the right leg and is in pain when the leg is moved. Her radiograph is shown:

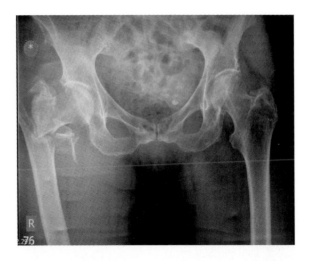

What type of fracture is this?

A. Intracapsular fracture of the right neck of femur
B. Intertrochanteric fracture of the right femur
C. Garden 2 fracture of the right neck of femur
D. Extracapsular fracture of the left neck of femur
E. Garden 4 fracture of the right neck of femur

Question 6

A 17-year-old boy who has lost control of his motorcycle at high speed attends A&E as a trauma call. The primary survey is normal. He complains of a painful left arm, the X-ray of which is shown:

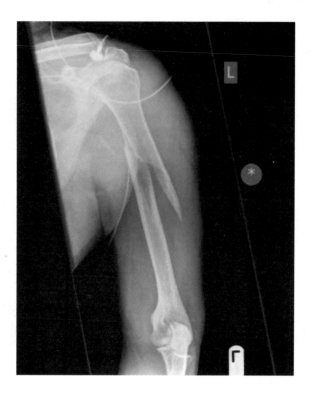

1. **What structure is in most danger as a result of this injury?**
A. Radial nerve
B. Median nerve
C. Ulnar nerve
D. Circumflex artery of the neck of humerus
E. The axillary artery

2. **How would you test for the integrity of the structure most at risk?**
A. Sensation over the upper deltoid
B. Extension at the wrist
C. Feel for the brachial pulse
D. Flex at the thumb
E. Abduct the fingers

Question 7

A 24-year-old man attends A&E after being tackled during a football match. He is unable to bend his knee and is in severe pain. There is an obvious swelling over the lateral knee joint which is hard to touch. His radiograph is shown below:

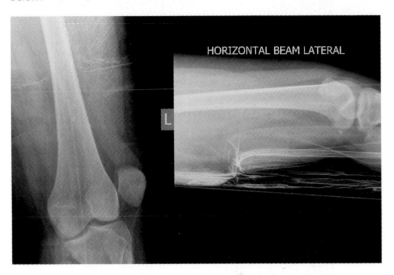

HORIZONTAL BEAM LATERAL

What is the diagnosis?
A. Fracture of the lateral condyle of the femur
B. Tibial plateau fracture
C. Dislocated patella
D. Distal femur fracture
E. No bony injuries but severe soft tissue injuries causing the swelling

Question 8

A builder falls to the ground from some scaffolding, from a height of 10 feet. He is taken to his local A&E and a trauma call is sounded. He is stabilised and the only injury he sustained is shown. The soft tissues are intact. An operation in the next few hours is planned and his limb is placed in a back slab. He is complaining of increasing pain in his right leg despite large doses of opiate analgesic agents and has now started to notice some numbness in his foot.

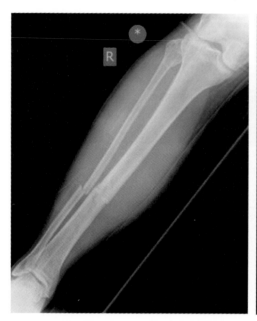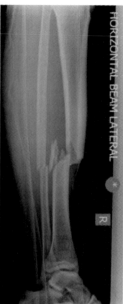

What is the major concern associated with this type of injury and the clinical picture?

A. Compartment syndrome

B. Nerve injury around the fracture site

C. Blood vessel injury around the fracture site

D. Undiagnosed spinal trauma

E. Anxiety and hysteria due to the injury

Question 9

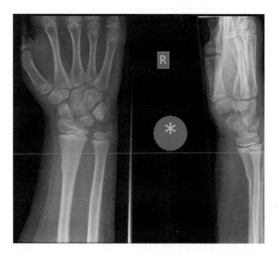

1. What age bracket does the patient with the above radiographs fall into? Justify your answer.
A. < 5 years
B. 5–15 years
C. 16–25 years
D. 23–35 years
E. > 40 years

This patient fell onto his outstretched right arm. He is complaining of very mild pain around the wrist joint but is able to move it relatively pain-free.

2. What do the above radiographs show?
A. No bony injury
B. Intra-articular fracture of the distal radius
C. Fracture of the distal third of the radius
D. Lunate dislocation
E. Scaphoid fracture

Question 10

A 16-year-old boy presents after being involved in a fight. He threw several punches and is now complaining of pain and swelling in his right hand. There is no soft tissue injury. His radiographs are shown below:

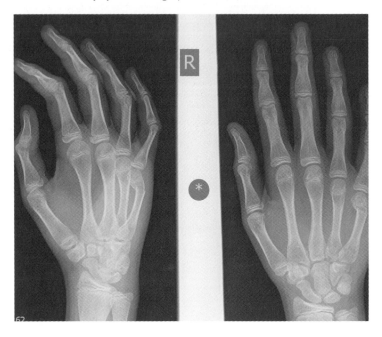

What do the radiographs show?

A. Fracture of the fifth metacarpal neck
B. Dislocation of the proximal interphalangeal joint of the fifth finger
C. Fracture of the waist of the scaphoid
D. Fracture of the third and fourth metacarpal necks
E. No bony injuries

Question 11

A child falls onto their left elbow and sustains a supracondylar fracture, as shown in the radiographs below:

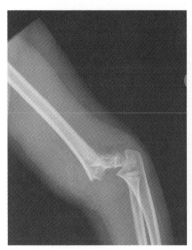 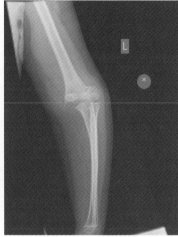

Which structure lying posterior to the condylar region is at risk?
A. Ulnar nerve
B. Radial nerve
C. Median nerve
D. Brachial artery
E. Basilic vein

Question 12

A 34-year-old man is involved in a road traffic accident. Primary and secondary trauma surveys reveal tenderness in his lower spine. A slice from a CT scan is shown.

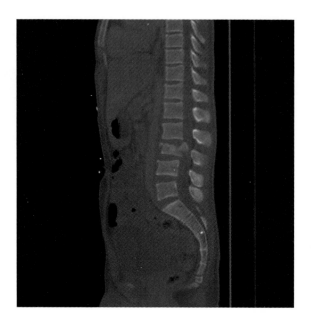

At what level is the most obvious bony injury which encroaches on the spinal canal?
A. L1
B. L2
C. L3
D. L4
E. L5

Question 13

A 54-year-old man slips on an icy pavement and lands on his left shoulder. He comes to A&E where a radiograph is taken. He has taken only paracetamol for pain relief. On examination, he is noted to have a loss of sensation over the lateral aspect of the left shoulder.

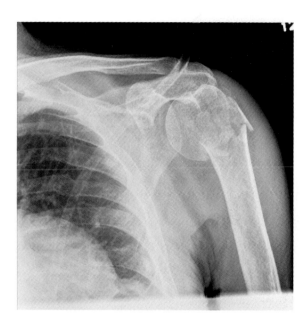

What is the most likely cause?
A. Damage to long thoracic nerve
B. Damage to the thoracodorsal nerve
C. Damage to the axillary nerve
D. Paraesthesia due to hypersensitivity to paracetamol
E. Damage to the circumflex arteries

Question 14

A 63-year-old man presents to A&E with a 3-day history of a swollen right knee. He has no history of trauma. He is able to fully weight-bear on his right leg and can flex the knee actively from 0 to 60 degrees. The A&E SHO aspirates the knee and obtains the following results:

Cloudy synovial fluid, 20,000 leucocytes/mm^3
No growth on cultures
Negatively birefringent needle-shaped crystals seen

What is the diagnosis?
A. Septic arthritis
B. Rheumatoid arthritis
C. Gout
D. Pseudogout
E. Osteoarthritis

Question 15

A 61-year-old woman presents to her GP complaining of long-standing pain and deformity in her hands. Her radiograph is shown below:

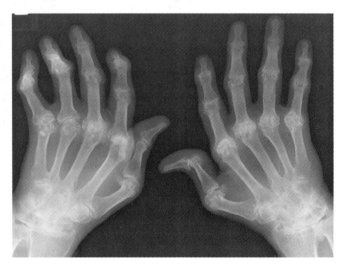

What is the most likely diagnosis?
A. Septic arthritis of the small joints of the hand
B. Rheumatoid arthritis
C. Psoriatic arthropathy
D. Polytrauma with evidence of malunion
E. Bony metastases

Question 16

A 46-year-old carpet layer presents to A&E complaining of a large swelling over his left knee (pictured). He is finding it difficult to kneel and is otherwise systemically well. On examination he has a large, warm and erythematous swelling over the left knee. He can actively fully flex his knee and it is relatively pain-free. His blood profile shows a normal white cell count and raised inflammatory markers. His radiograph is also shown below.

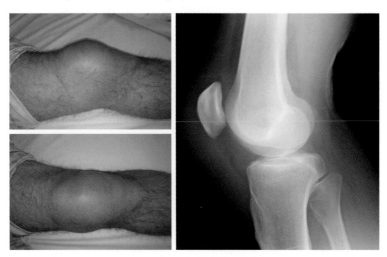

What is the diagnosis?
A. Septic arthritis
B. Cellulitis of the lower limb
C. Ruptured Baker's cyst
D. Ligamentous and meniscal injury
E. Pre-patellar bursitis

Question 17

A 14-year-old boy is brought to A&E complaining of right groin pain. On examination, he has a limp, with difficulty weight-bearing, and there is external rotation of the right lower limb. Hip movements are restricted and painful. He has no other medical history. His radiographs are shown:

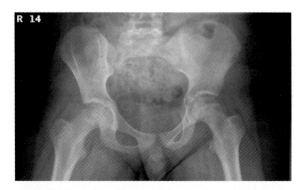

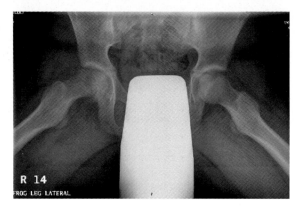

What is the diagnosis?
A. Fractured right neck of femur
B. Right hip dislocation
C. Perthes' disease
D. Slipped upper femoral epiphysis
E. Soft tissue trauma

Question 18

A 67-year-old male patient, with a known malignancy, is sent for a bone isotope scan after complaining of generalised body pain. The scan is shown and highlights multiple bone deposits.

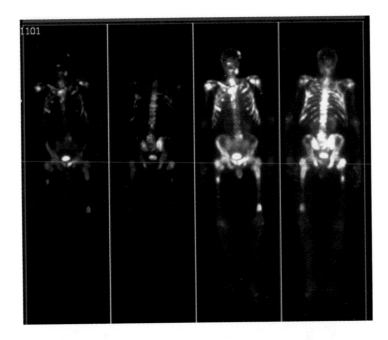

What are the five common primary malignancies which commonly metastasise to bone?
A. Breast, renal, lung, prostate, parotid
B. Breast, renal, lung, bowel, thyroid
C. Breast, renal, lung, bowel, liver
D. Breast, renal, lung, prostate, thyroid
E. Breast, liver, lung, prostate, thyroid

Question 19

A 33-year-old man attends A&E after hurting his shoulder whilst playing rugby. He is in significant pain and is unwilling to move at the shoulder joint. There is no neurovascular deficit to the left upper limb. His radiographs are shown:

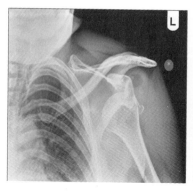 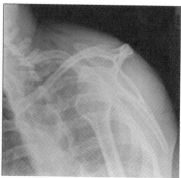

What is the diagnosis?

A. Anterior dislocation of the shoulder
B. Fracture of the lateral clavicle
C. Fracture of the scapula
D. Acromioclavicular joint dislocation
E. Fracture of the left humeral head

Question 20

A 63-year-old man presents to clinic complaining of intermittent swelling in his knee. He is able to weight bear but he can find this uncomfortable. On examination there is a knee effusion but there is no erythema and the knee is not warm to touch. He is able to actively flex the knee from 0 to 80 degrees with mild discomfort. His radiograph is shown:

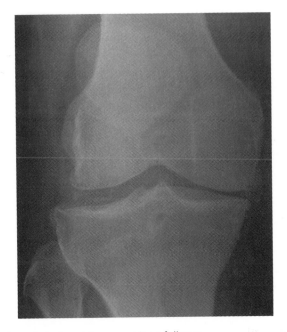

His knee is aspirated and the report is as follows:
Cloudy synovial fluid
Few white cells
No growth on culture
Positively birefrigent rhomboid shaped crystals seen

1. What is the diagnosis?
A. Septic arthritis
B. Rheumatoid arthritis
C. Gout
D. Pseudogout
E. Osteoarthritis

2. What feature of the above condition is shown in the radiograph?
A. Osteophytes
B. Loss of joint space
C. Chondrocalcinosis
D. Subchondral sclerosis
E. Bony cysts

Musculoskeletal Medicine and Trauma

Answers

Question 1

B Volar displacement of the distal radius

The radiograph shows the classical Colles' fracture. It is an extra-articular fracture of the distal radius. The displacement of the distal radius is dorsal, not volar. The other features are shortening of the radius and radial tilt. It is sometimes referred to as a 'dinner fork deformity', as the clinical deformity resembles a dinner fork when viewed laterally.

Question 2

1. C Distal fibula fracture (Weber B) and subluxation of the ankle joint

This unfortunate lady has sustained several injuries to her ankle. She has an obvious fracture to her distal fibula and a subluxation of her ankle joint. The Weber classification system, described below, uses the position of the distal tibiofibular ligaments or syndesmosis to classify the fracture. This is a type B. You may also notice a tiny bony chip between the medial malleolus and the talus, representing an avulsion fracture at that site.

Weber classification of ankle fractures	
Type A	Fracture below the level of the tibiofibular syndesmotic ligament
Type B	Fracture at level of the joint, with the tibiofibular syndesmotic ligaments usually intact
Type C	Fracture above the joint level which commonly disrupts the syndesmotic ligaments

2. D *Closed reduction and immobilise in plaster back slab and elevation*

The principles of management of any fracture are the 4 Rs: resuscitation – reduction – restriction (i.e. immobilisation) – rehabilitation. This fracture and the subluxation of the joint need to be reduced to help with both the pain and the soft tissue swelling. These injuries are usually acutely immobilised in a plaster 'back slab'; full casts may be applied but should be split so that the cast has 'give' to accommodate increases in swelling and to avoid rises in compartment pressure due to tight casts.

Question 3

D *Varus deformity of the knee*

Although joint and limb deformity may occur in advanced cases of osteoarthritis, the deformity does not have to be varus. The other features are the classic radiological features of osteoarthritis and should be memorised as they are frequently asked about in examinations.

Question 4

B *Hemiarthroplasty of the right hip*

This woman has sustained a right-sided intracapsular neck of femur fracture. These types of fracture can be easily classified using the Garden classification (outlined below). This is a displaced fracture. Type 1 and 2 may be treated using screws, whereas types 3 and 4 usually require replacement of the femoral head as the blood supply to it is likely to have been disrupted. In younger or more active patients, a total hip replacement rather than a hemiarthroplasty may be more appropriate surgical treatment.

(Remember the mnemonic 1-2-Screw, 3-4 Austin Moore)

Garden classification for neck of femur fractures	
Garden type 1	Incomplete/valgus impacted
Garden type 2	Undisplaced, complete
Garden type 3	Complete fracture, partially displaced
Garden type 4	Complete fracture, completely displaced (trabecular pattern of head assumes orientation parallel to acetabulum)

Question 5

B *Intertrochanteric fracture of the right femur*

This is an extracapsular, intertrochanteric fracture of the right hip. The intertrochanteric line joins the greater and lesser trochanter of the proximal femur. Both trochanters are also fractured (four-part fracture). The Garden classification is used for intracapsular fractures of the neck of femur, but this injury is extracapsular. This fracture can be treatment by using a dynamic hip screw or an intramedullary hip screw device

Question 6

1. A *Radial nerve*

This young man has sustained a displaced, oblique fracture through the midshaft of his left humerus. Many structures are at risk, however the structure we are most concerned about is the radial nerve, which runs in the spiral groove on the posterior aspect of the mid-humerus. Obviously all the other structures must also be assessed.

2. B *Extension at the wrist*

The easiest way to assess an injury to the radial nerve at the level of the mid-arm is to ask the patient to extend his or her wrist. However, it is important that a full and detailed assessment of all the structures and movement listed in the question is done.

Question 7

C *Dislocated patella*

The radiographs show a dislocated patella. On the anteroposterior (AP) view, the patella is clearly displaced laterally, which is the commonest direction in which it dislocates. On the lateral view, it is apparent that the patella is not sitting in its normal position anterior to the knee joint. This injury tends to be a clinical diagnosis and can usually be reduced back to its anatomical position in A&E.

Question 8

A *Compartment syndrome*

The major concern in this scenario is that of a developing compartment syndrome. The musculature of the leg is divided into four compartments surrounded by tight fascia. When the long bones are fractured, the soft tissues begin to swell in their fascial compartments. This can lead to raised pressures within the compartments. If not recognised and treated promptly it may lead to muscle ischaemia and tissue death.

Question 9

1. B *5–15 years*
By observing the radiographs, we can clear see non-fused growth plates. This means that they are of a young patient (i.e. an immature skeleton). However, the appearance of all the ossific nuclei of the carpal bones means that this patient is likely to be older than 5 years.

2. C *Fracture of the distal third of the radius*
The radiograph shows a buckle or torus fracture of the distal radius. Children's bones are yet to mineralise fully and as a result are 'softer' than adult bones. This means that they have a tendency to bend rather than break, but this is still a fracture! Notice the subtle 'swelling' and irregularity of both cortices at the distal radius in the AP view (see arrows in radiographs below). The step in the distal radius is more obvious in the lateral view. This can be treated conservatively in a plaster cast as it will heal and remodel fully.

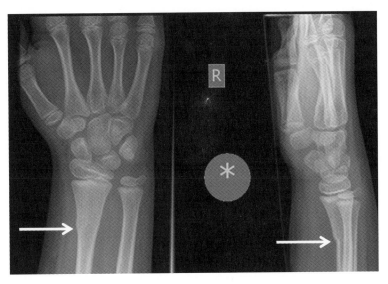

Question 10

A Fracture of the fifth metacarpal neck

The radiographs show an angulated fracture of the fifth metacarpal neck. This is commonly a punch injury and is often referred to as a Boxer's fracture.

Question 11

A Ulnar nerve

The ulnar nerve runs posteriorly to the medial epicondyle and is clearly at risk in this injury. However, this is clearly a high-energy injury and, as such, the other structures listed may also have been damaged. The brachial artery is at risk as it is stretched across the front of the distal humerus fracture and the anterior interosseous nerve is the most commonly injured nerve. Hence it is imperative that a detailed neurovascular examination is conducted, documented and repeated regularly, both before and after the fracture is taken to theatre, reduced and stabilised.

Question 12

C L3

This is an easy question to answer if you know that there are five lumbar vertebrae. Start counting backwards from above the sacrum. Remember, the spinal column in an adult ends at L1/L2. Below this level it continues as the cauda equina. From the MRI we can see an obvious fracture involving L3 and a possible injury to the anterior L4 vertebral body.

Question 13

C Damage to the axillary nerve

The axillary nerve wraps itself around the surgical neck of the humerus. Thus it is susceptible to damage when the neck is fractured, as shown in the radiograph. The axillary nerve supplies two muscles (deltoid, teres minor) and sensation to the skin over the lateral aspect of the shoulder region. With an acute fracture, it may be difficult to assess power of these muscles but sensation is easy to assess over the upper shoulder (regimental badge area).

Question 14

C *Gout*

Swollen knees are a very common reason for people to seek medical attention. Septic arthritis needs to be recognised and excluded as soon as possible. Aspiration involves removing some intra-articular synovial fluid from the joint via a needle using an aseptic technique. Samples are then sent for microscopy, culture and crystal analysis.

In the absence of significantly raised white cells on haematology and organisms on microscopy or culture, septic arthritis can usually be excluded.

A diagnosis of gout can be confirmed by the presence of negatively birefringent, needle-shaped monosodium urate crystals. Weakly positive rhomboid shaped calcium pyrophosphate crystals are found in pseudogout.

Osteoarthritis is usually a radiographic diagnosis and may coexist with the other diagnoses.

Question 15

B *Rheumatoid arthritis*

There is clearly evidence of extensive small joint inflammatory arthritis in both hands. Note the deformity of her fingers and thumbs, especially the characteristic Z- thumbs and ulnar deviation of her fingers.

Question 16

E *Pre-patellar bursitis*

Also known as 'housemaid's knee' this condition tends to affect people who kneel down whilst they work. The patient is able to flex his knee and may still be relatively pain-free, which makes septic arthritis less likely. The photograph shows a tense extra-articular swelling superficial to the patella with some overlying erythema. The radiograph also shows a large swelling anterior to the patella, but the joint itself does not have an effusion. Remember that when in doubt, one can attempt to aspirate the knee but care must be taken not to attempt this through infected skin as this may actually introduce infection into a non-infected joint.

This is an inflammatory bursitis – the WCC is likely to be normal and it is treated with anti-inflammatories, elevation and avoidance of the activity which precipitates it (i.e. kneeling). A bursitis may be infected, especially after breaks in the skin and may need antibiotics and surgical drainage.

Question 17

D *Slipped upper femoral epiphysis*
This boy has suffered a slipped upper femoral epiphysis (SUFE). This is evident in the AP radiograph of the pelvis, however it is much clearer in the 'frog's leg view' radiograph (see arrows in radiograph below).

This condition is a common cause for hip or knee pain (referred pain from the hip) in adolescents. It can rarely occur after a traumatic event, but most children do not recall any trauma. In the growing skeleton the cartilage epiphyseal plate (physis) is weaker than the surrounding bone. Overweight children can be more prone to developing SUFE.

The main cause of SUFE is likely to be from an increased shear force on the hip at a time when the head of the femur is unable to support these forces. The femoral head fails through the physis (the weakest point). Consequently, a condition similar to a stress fracture develops. Surgical fixation is usually required to prevent further slippage of the epiphysis.

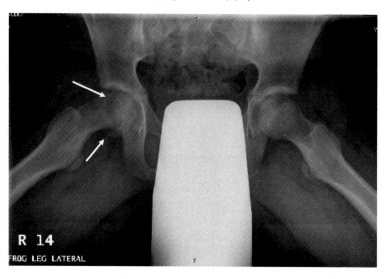

Question 18

D Breast, renal, lung, prostate, thyroid

Although all cancers have the potential to metastasise to bone, the five common malignancies are: thyroid, lung, breast, renal, prostate. An easy way to remember this is to image a hexagon on a torso; each point refers to one of the five common sites (see diagram below). Or if you prefer mnemonics: BLT with Ketchup and Pickle!

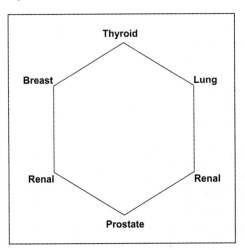

Question 19

A Anterior dislocation of the shoulder

This is a common injury scenario seen in A&E. The radiographs clearly show that the humerus is dislocated and is not in contact with the glenoid. Anterior dislocations are more common than posterior ones. This should be reduced in A&E under sedation. It is vital to assess the neurovascular status of the limb both pre- and post-reduction.

Question 20

1. D Pseudogout

From the aspirate result, the diagnosis is pseudogout. See the answer to Question 14 for a more detailed explanation

2. C *Chondrocalcinosis*

One of the radiological features of pseudogout is chondrocalcinosis: calcification of the cartilage within a joint. This is shown by the arrows in the radiograph below. The other features mentioned in the question are, of course, the radiological features of osteoarthritis. Calcium pyrophosphate dehydrate deposition can take several forms as a clinical entity. Asymptomatic chondrocalcinosis is common in elderly patients and is seen in association with osteoarthritis. It can also present as an acute synovitis (pseudogout) or a chronic pyrophosphate arthropathy.

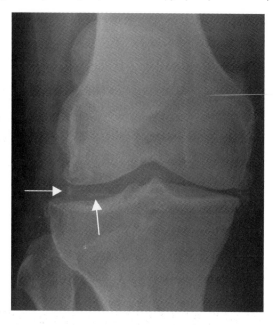

8 Dermatology

Questions

Claudia Carmaciu and Rohaj Mehta

Question 1

A 27-year-old patient presents to his GP complaining of asymmetrical hair loss. He noticed months ago that his hair was falling out in patches.

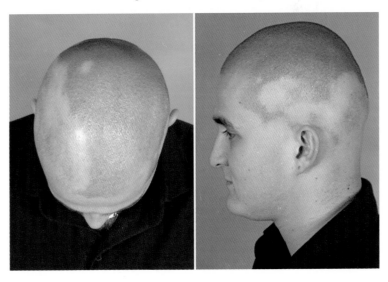

Clinical Data Interpretation for Medical Finals: Single Best Answer Questions, First Edition.
Edited by Philip Socrates Pastides and Parveen Jayia.
© 2012 Philip Socrates Pastides and Parveen Jayia. Published 2012 by John Wiley & Sons, Ltd.

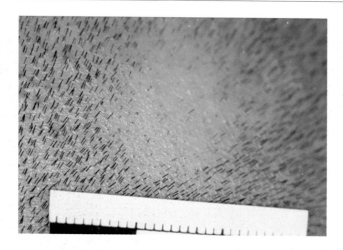

What is the most likely diagnosis?
A. Alopecia areata
B. Early-onset male pattern baldness
C. Tinea corporis
D. Vitiligo
E. Alopecia totalis

Question 2

A 31-year-old woman is admitted with abdominal pain. She is also noted to have a generalised purpuric rash, predominantly on the lower limbs. She has no significant medical history but mentions having been treated for a sore throat by her GP last week.

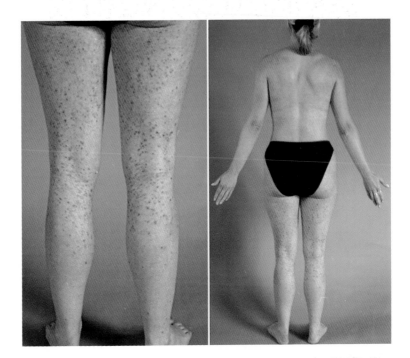

What is the most likely diagnosis?

A. Hereditary haemorrhagic telangiectasia
B. Henoch–Schönlein purpura
C. Measles
D. Erythroderma
E. Guttate psoriasis

Question 3

A 76-year-old woman presents to her GP with the lesion in the photographs. She has had it for several years and it has not changed in appearance.

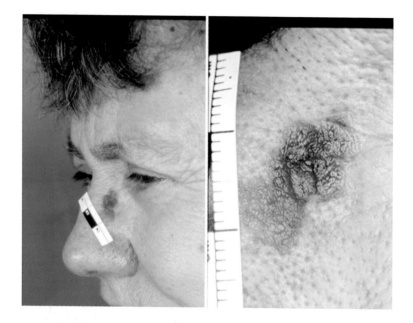

What is the most likely diagnosis?

A. Melanoma

B. Seborrhoeic wart

C. Basal cell carcinoma

D. Squamous cell carcinoma

E. Keratin horn

Question 4

A 68-year-old man presents with the lesion shown. It is lying anterior to his left ear and has been growing rapidly over the past 4 weeks.

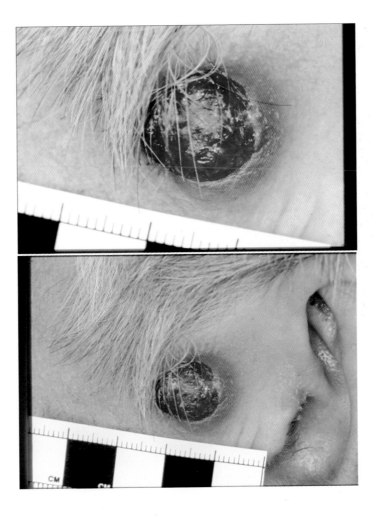

What is the most likely diagnosis?
1. Basal cell carcinoma
2. Keratocanthoma
3. Melanoma
4. Keloid scar
5. Orf

Question 5

A 26-year-old keen runner presents to his GP complaining of unsightly nails on his left foot. He says that initially only one nail was affected, but now it seems to be spreading to adjacent toenails.

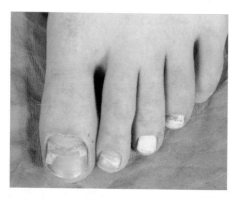

What is the most likely diagnosis?
A. Leukonychia totalis
B. Onychomycosis
C. Paronychia
D. Yellow nail syndrome
E. Trauma

Question 6

A 72-year-old man presents to his GP with a rough pink patch of skin on the left aspect of his nasal bridge. It is not bothersome and he is otherwise well, but his wife is concerned that he may have skin cancer.

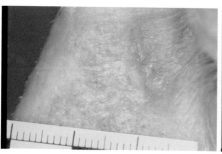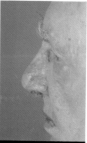

What is the most likely diagnosis?
1. Keratin horn
2. Eczema
3. Actinic keratosis
4. Basal cell carcinoma
5. Actinic elastosis

Question 7

A 50-year-old Australian nurse visits her GP on the advice of her husband, who is very concerned about a mole that appears to be changing.

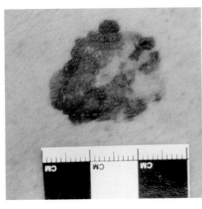
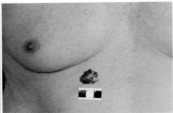

Which of the following criteria is not considered to be a clinical feature of melanoma:
A. Asymmetry
B. Border irregularity
C. Colour variegation
D. Diameter > 6 mm
E. Scaly surface

Question 8

A patient with malignant melanoma has the lesion excised and it is submitted for histopathological examination.

Which of the following is used as a prognostic factor in melanoma of the skin?
A. Dukes staging
B. Ann Arbor staging
C. FIGO system
D. Breslow's depth
E. NYHA classification

Question 9

A 28-year-old homeless man presents to the local walk-in clinic complaining of weight loss, night sweats and a cough over the past 3 months. Whilst examining the patient, the doctor finds some tender and firm reddish blue nodules over his shins.

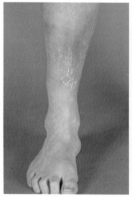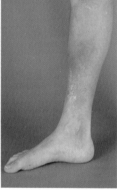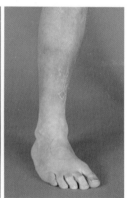

1. What is the most likely diagnosis?
A. Erythema multiforme
B. Erythema nodosum
C. Necrobiosis lipoidica
D. Sweet's disease
E. Dermatomyositis

2. Which of the following is least likely to be the cause of his rash?

A. Sulphonamides
B. Sarcoidosis
C. Tuberculosis
D. Inflammatory bowel disease
E. Bronchial carcinoma

Question 10

A 67-year-old man presents to his GP with a solitary asymptomatic lesion that he mentions has been enlarging over the past 2 years.

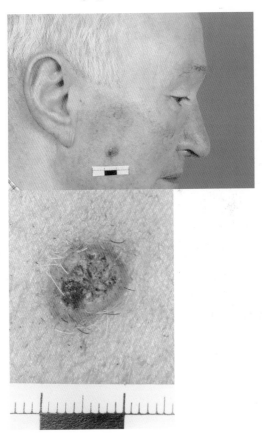

What is the most likely diagnosis?
A. Squamous cell carcinoma
B. Dermatofibroma
C. Melanoma
D. Basal cell carcinoma
E. Neurofibroma

Question 11

A 29-year-old professional cyclist presents with a well-circumscribed rash of varying hyperpigmented patches that have coalesced across his upper torso.

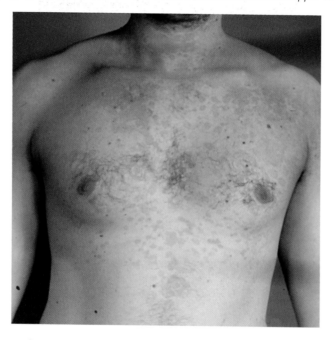

What is the most likely diagnosis?
A. Tinea corporis
B. Tinea manuum
C. Tinea cruris
D. Pityriasis versicolor
E. Tinea incognito

Question 12

A 92-year-old woman is an in-patient being treated for community-acquired pneumonia. A few days into her hospital stay she becomes febrile and develops an exfoliative rash over her whole body which is hot to the touch. She has no past medical history of skin conditions. Other than the antibiotics that were commenced on this admission, she takes no other medication.

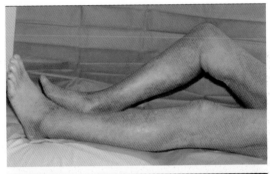

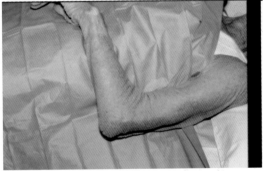

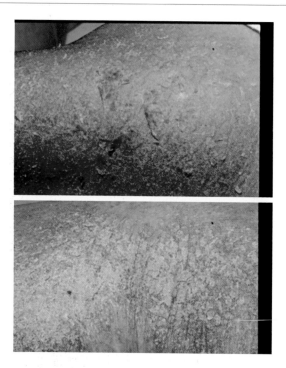

What is the most likely diagnosis?

A. Erythroderma
B. Toxic epidermal necrolysis
C. Erythema nodosum
D. Erythema multiforme
E. Scarlet fever

Question 13

A 45-year-old businesswoman is referred to the dermatologist due to flushing of the skin and persistence of papules and pustules across her cheeks, nose and forehead.

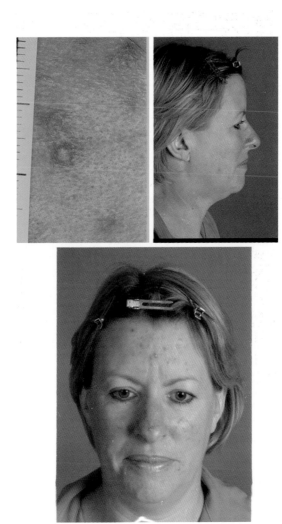

What is the most likely diagnosis?

A. Rosacea

B. Impetigo

C. Eczema

D. Systemic lupus erythematosus

E. Acne

Question 14

A 28-year-old woman presents with an all-over body rash that began with the one larger patch on the lower left of the abdomen. She mentions that she had a nasty cold and sore throat 1 week prior to the rash developing. The rash is non-pruritic and she is otherwise fit and well.

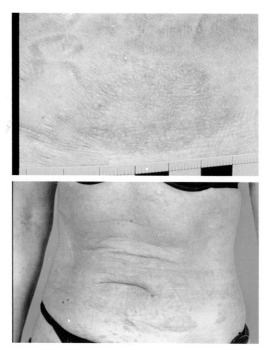

What is the most likely diagnosis?
A. Shingles
B. Measles
C. Chicken pox
D. Pityriasis rosea
E. Ringworm

Question 15

A 29-year-old builder comes to his GP with well-demarcated scaly plaques present on his elbows and knees. He is feeling increasingly self conscious at work because his colleagues won't share tools with him, claiming that they don't want to catch his disease.

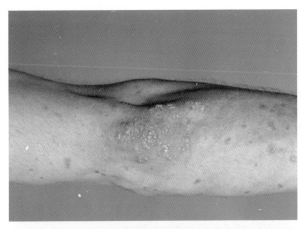

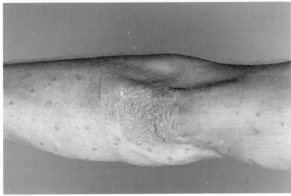

1. What is the most likely diagnosis?

A. Eczema

B. Psoriasis

C. Tinea corporis

D. Seborrhoeic dermatitis

E. Cellulitis

2. Which of the following is not a treatment for the condition?

A. PUVA

B. Vitamin D analogues

C. Methotrexate

D. Pethanol

E. UVB

Question 16

A 45-year-old woman comes to see her GP complaining of recurrent epistaxis. The GP notices a non blanching rash (see photographs below). The patient states she has had this for many years and several of her siblings also have the same condition.

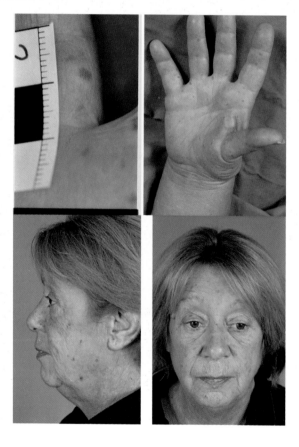

What is the most likely diagnosis?
A. Peutz–Jeghers Syndrome
B. Haemangioma
C. Hereditary haemorrhagic telangiectasia
D. Meningitis
E. Vasculitis

Question 17

A 70-year-old retired farmer presents to his GP with a lesion that has been growing over the past 6 months.

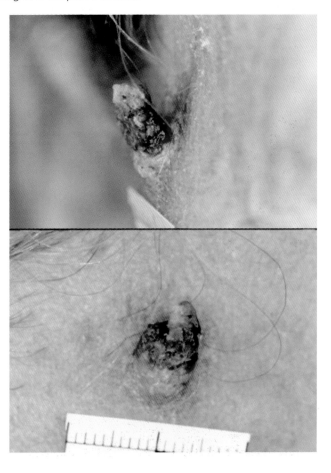

Which one of the following is correct for the lesion shown above?

A. Occasionally have malignant lesions at their base

B. It is the most common skin cancer

C. More frequent in those aged < 50 years

D. Never found on hands or feet

E. It is composed of compacted groups of large melanocytes

Question 18

A 45-year-old man with hypothyroidism presents to his GP with the rash seen below. It is painless, non-itchy and has been present for the past 4 months.

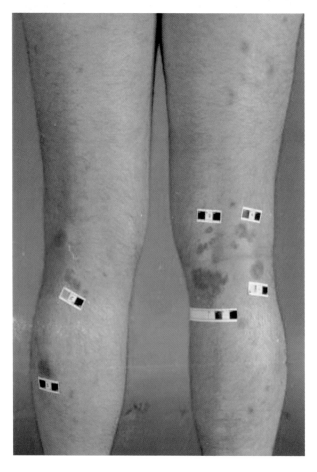

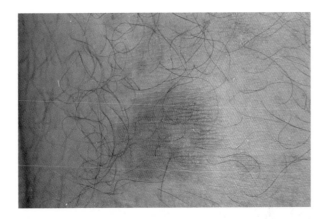

1. Which condition best fits the presentation and image shown?
A. Tinea corporis
B. Granuloma annulare
C. Eczema
D. Erythema nodosum
E. Necrobiosis lipoidica

2. What is the most suitable option for treatment?
A. Antifungals
B. Antibiotics
C. No treatment required
D. Tar-impregnated bandages
E. Excision

Dermatology

Answers

Question 1

A *Alopecia areata*

Alopecia areata occurs when the anagen phase (this is the growing phase in the hair cycle) is arrested. The exact cause is unknown, but genetics, autoimmune disease and stress are commonly associated.

The age of onset is typically the second or third decade. The symptoms consist of small, smooth, bald patches that are usually round in shape. It most often affects the scalp, resulting in patchy (areata) or total (totalis) scalp hair loss. It can rarely result in the loss of all bodily hair (universalis). The pattern may be asymmetrical, so one side of the scalp can be affected more than the other.

Another pathognomonic feature is the presence of exclamation mark hairs. This refers to hair that becomes narrower along the length of the strand towards the base. Patients with alopecia may also notice that their hair pulls out much more easily.

The course and pattern are unpredictable but regrowth after a first presentation is common. Localised disease may spontaneously resolve and may be aided by the use of intralesional steroid injections. Extensive disease is more difficult to treat and associated with a poorer outcome.

Aside from treating the hair loss, it is important that the psychological aspect of the condition is managed, mainly those of psychosocial issues relating to body image, social phobia, anxiety and depression.

Other causes of hair loss include androgenetic alopecia (male pattern baldness), infections (ringworm), trauma and traction (pulling tightly at hair), burns, endocrine disease (such as hypo/hyperthyroidism) and malnutrition (iron/zinc/protein deficiency).

Question 2

B *Henoch–Schönlein purpura*

Henoch–Schönlein purpura (HSP) is an IgA-mediated autoimmune systemic condition. The purpura typically appears on the legs and buttocks, but may also be seen on the arms, face and trunk. It is most common in childhood and is usually preceded by a streptococcal infection such as pharyngitis.

Aside from the rash, there is a classic triad of arthralgia, abdominal pain and haematuria. The most worrying complication is that of acute kidney injury. Henoch–Schönlein nephritis is indistinguishable from that of IgA nephropathy, characteristically showing a focal and segmental proliferative glomerulonephritis. This may result in permanent and chronic kidney damage.

Diagnosis is made on clinical grounds and supported by blood tests which may show kidney function derangement, raised IgA levels and inflammatory markers. It is usually a self-limiting condition that requires close monitoring of systemic function and supportive treatment.

Question 3

B *Seborrhoeic wart*
Seborrhoeic warts (basal cell papillomas) are the most common benign tumours of the elderly and are due to benign proliferation of epidermal cells which result in the characteristic 'stuck on' appearance.

They are often multiple, enlarge with time and become darkly pigmented. Dermoscopy can be useful to distinguish these lesions from melanocytic lesions, and if there is still doubt then a biopsy can be taken and treatment would be to curette them.

Treatment is not usually necessary but sometimes they can catch on clothes and jewellery, so in this case they can be curetted or treated with cryotherapy.

Question 4

B *Keratocanthoma*
Keratocanthoma is a rapidly growing solitary lesion that progresses to a dome-shaped nodule with a shiny surface, leading to crater formation with a keratin plug and finally self-resolving within 3 months, often leaving an unsightly scar.

It pathologically resembles squamous cell carcinoma (SCC). Some keratocanthomas arise from an SCC, whilst other keratocanthomas go on to develop into an SCC, therefore treatment in the first instance should be by excision where possible.

Causes include both sunlight (these lesions arise most commonly in sun-exposed areas of the body) and chemical carcinogens. Human papilloma virus, genetic factors, trauma and immunocompromised status have also been implicated as contributory factors.

Orfs are common in medical school exams. They are solitary papules that become painful purple pustules with an umbilicated centre, generally found on the hand (and in exams, the hands of farmer's wives!). They occur as a result of a pox virus that is endemic in sheep.

Question 5

B Onychomycosis (fungal nail infection)

Fungal infection of the nails is common, particularly in those with tinea pedis (athlete's foot). Onychomycosis is more commonly seen on the feet than on the hands.

The infection often begins at the distal nail edge and extends proximally, eventually involving the whole nail (as seen in the middle toe). The nail thickens, separates from the nail bed and becomes very fragile and crumbly.

Treatment is not advised unless nail clippings have been sent, confirming the diagnosis. Thereafter, treatment involves oral antifungals (e.g. terbinafine) for up to 6 months or more depending on the rate of nail regrowth.

- Leukonychia totalis – whitening of the entire nail due to hypoalbuminaemia
- Paronychia – painful boggy swelling of lateral/proximal nail fold, expelling pus when pressure is applied, commonly due to bacteria (*Staphylococcus/Streptococcus*) and requiring treatment with antibiotics
- Yellow nail syndrome – rare medical condition that is common in exams! Triad of pleural effusions, lymphoedema and dystrophic yellow nails.

Question 6

C Actinic (solar) keratosis

Actinic keratosis may present as single or multiple scaly lesions. They classically feel rough (like sandpaper) to the touch and are commonly found on sun-exposed areas in persons of older age. They may occasionally regress spontaneously, however actinic keratosis can progress to SCC.

Treatment is normally by cryosurgery, although topical application of 5% fluorouracil cream is also an option. Cutaneous (keratin) horns may develop over the top and thus require excision.

Actinic elastosis is yellow, thickened and wrinkled skin, common in those that work outdoors.

Question 7

E Scaly surface

Melanoma is a malignant cancer of the melanocytes of the skin. The incidence is more frequent in women and among the Caucasian population living in sunny climates. Repeated short bursts of exposure to ultraviolet radiation (e.g. sunbeds), having multiple melanocytic naevi, a positive family history of melanoma and atypical mole syndrome (ATMS) are known risk factors.

This is **a common** exam question. Recognising melanomas in exams is not difficult if a pattern is followed. Try using the following mnemonic, ABCDE:

- **A**symmetrical lesion
- **B**orders that are irregular
- **C**olour changes within the lesion
- **D**iameter that changes and is > 6 mm
- **E**volving or **E**nlarging lesions

Other features include a pruritic lesion that may bleed easily and the presence of satellite lesions. If any of these features are seen, urgent referral to a dermatologist is needed.

Management involves surgical excision and histopathological examination. Prognosis relates to depth of the tumour. Prevention and early recognition are key. This is done through education of the public regarding importance of preventing excessive sun exposure and recognising the need to report changes in a mole to a health professional.

Question 8

D *Breslow's depth*

Breslow's depth is used as a prognostic indicator for melanomas. It is determined using an ocular micrometer to directly measure the depth to which the tumour cells have invaded the skin. Measurement is taken from the granular layer of the epidermis down to the deepest point of invasion. This measurement has been shown to accurately predict the risk for lymph node metastasis and provides us with an approximate 5-year survival rate.

Breslow thickness	Approximate 5-year survival
< 1 mm	95–100%
1–2 mm	80–96%
2.1–4 mm	60–75%
> 4 mm	50%

The other staging tools are used in the following:
- Dukes staging – colon cancer
- Ann Arbor staging – lymphoma
- FIGO staging – ovarian cancer
- NYHA classification – heart failure

Question 9

1. B *Erythema nodosum*

Erythema nodosum is a panniculitis. This simply means inflammation of the subcutaneous adipose tissue, presenting most commonly as red, firm and tender nodules over the lower legs. Panniculitis can be caused by cold or trauma. Both are possible in this patient's case, however the added history should make you suspicious of erythema nodosum. If there is a cough, night sweats and weight loss, think of tuberculosis (TB)!

Erythema nodosum is believed to be due to a delayed hypersensitivity reaction to a wide variety of antigens. The most common causes in exams are TB, sarcoidosis and inflammatory bowel disease (IBD).

The nodules heal spontaneously and 20% of patients have idiopathic erythema nodosum. However, as this condition can be due to more serious underlying disease- it is important to investigate the patient thoroughly to exclude other pathology.

Below is a list of the more common causes and appropriate investigations:

Causes	Investigations
Bacterial infections	
Streptococcal	Blood cultures, throat swab (group A β-hameolytic strep), ASO[a]
Tuberculosis	Chest X-ray, Mantoux test
Leprosy	Sexual and travel history
Salmonella, Campylobacter	History of any gastrointestinal complaints and stool cultures if appropriate
Drugs	
Sulphonamides	i.e. sulfamethoxazole (component of co-trimoxazole = trimethoprim, a commonly used antibacterial for urinary tract infections), furosemide (diuretic), sumatriptan (for migraines)
Oral contraceptives	
Sarcoidosis	Chest X-ray (classically showing bilateral hilar lymphadenopathy), serum Ca^{2+} ↑, urine Ca^{2+} ↑, serum angiotensin-converting enzyme (ACE)↑
Inflammatory bowel disease	History of gastrointestinal complaints Investigation for ulcerative colitis/Crohn's disease (colonoscopy and biopsy)
Cancer	Lymphoma, Leukaemia

[a] Anti-streptolysin titre (ASO) = blood test for antibodies produced against streptococcus, indicating past/present infection.

2. E *Bronchial carcinoma*

Bronchial carcinoma is not a documented cause of erythema nodosum.

Question 10

D *Basal cell carcinoma*

Basal cell carcinoma (BCCs) are the most common skin cancer. They arise from the basal keratinocytes of the epidermis and, although locally invasive (hence the common name of 'rodent ulcer'), they rarely metastasise.

The majority of BCCs occur on sun-exposed skin and in fair-skinned patients. Prolonged exposure to UV light is known to induce malignant transformation of basal cells and so is a causative factor in BCCs.

The classical appearance and description of BCCs in exams is a pearly papule with fine telangiectasia. Central necrosis may occur, leaving a small ulcer with an overlying crust.

Management depends on size and location of the BCC. Ideally complete excision is the best treatment. However, if this is not possible then confirmation by biopsy followed by radiotherapy is suitable for older patients. Those on the face require specialist management.

The majority of cases are treated before any serious complications arise. However, if these rodent ulcers are left untreated, they can destroy surrounding soft tissue, cartilage and even bone.

You would be forgiven for mistaking a BCC for a SCC on appearance alone, but the latter are usually more rapidly growing, bleed more easily and some ulcerated BCCs can also be associated with a foul smell.

Clues can be found in the patient information provided; i.e. in SCC the exam question may mention the lesion to arise from a scar, on the lips or in the mucosa (these are the more common sites for aggressive ulcerating forms of SCC). Also, SCCs are more common in immunosuppressed patients (i.e. HIV).

Nevertheless, these are exam tips and in the clinical setting these lesions would ideally all be excised and diagnosis confirmed histopathologically.

Question 11

D *Pityriasis versicolor*

Pityriasis versicolor is a common fungal infection of the skin often caused by *Malassezia furfur* (a component of normal skin flora). The rash can be either hyperpigmented (as seen in the image in the question) or hypopigmented, and often reveals a variance in skin hue (hence the name versicolor = variance in colour).

This is especially obvious if the person has had recent excessive exposure to sunlight, as the patches where there is overgrowth of the fungus do not tan. The classic exam question is one of a patient recently back from holiday, who presents with pale patches over the torso.

Treatment is usually with antifungal creams or shampoos used to wash the whole body. Patients must be reassured that the discoloration may persist until their suntan has gone!

Tinea corporis is another common fungal skin infection comprising single or multiple scaly plaques that are well demarcated and circular (hence the term 'ringworm', which leads to the common misconception that this infection is caused by a worm). The commonest causative organisms include *Tricophyton verrucosum, Tricophyton rubrum* and *Microsporum canis*.

Other superficial fungal infections include tinea captitis (of the head), tinea cruris (in the groin region), tinea manuum (of the hand) and tinea pedis (athlete's foot).

Tinea incognitio is a fungal infection caused by a topical immunosuppressive agent, i.e. steroid use.

Treatment of fungal skin infections is made up of three parts:

1. Avoidance of humid and sweaty conditions
2. Topical therapy (antifungal cream, such as clotrimazole or anti-fungal all-over-body washes)
3. Systemic therapy (oral antifungals).

Remember that antifungals may be hepatotoxic, so patients need liver function tests when taking oral medication.

Do not forget that ringworm is infectious. Therefore care must be taken in gyms not to walk barefoot and towels should not be shared by other family members.

Question 12

A *Erythroderma*

Erythroderma is a dermatological emergency. It is a generalized exfoliative dermatitis involving the majority of the skin surface and often occurs as a result of already existing dermatosis or systemic disease. In a third of patients, the cause is a reaction to drugs (such as antibiotics in this patient example).

The more common causes of erythroderma are as follows:

- Eczema
- Psoriasis
- Lymphoma/Sezary syndrome
- Drug reactions

The term 'red man syndrome' is commonly used for erythroderma. Features that are common to all patients with erythroderma include a patchy erythema that quickly spreads. Other features include pyrexia and rigors. The skin is hot to the touch and very red. This leads to heat loss and hypothermia, resulting in an increased basal metabolic rate. Fluid loss is excessively transpired and the resulting clinical picture is similar to that seen in patients with burns (hypoalbuminaemia, cutaneous oedema, dehydration and finally cardiac failure).

It is important to realise that the erythrodermic patient is susceptible to secondary infection. Management is supportive. Emollients and topical steroids can be useful.

Toxic epidermal necrolysis (TEN), which occurs as a reaction to drugs, also presents with red swollen skin. In TEN the skin shears in response to light pressure (Nikolsky sign) due to separation of skin layers at the basement membrane. This is different from the flaky exfoliative appearance of erythroderma, seen in the images.

Question 13

A *Rosacea*

Rosacea is a chronic condition, characterized by erythema of the skin (particularly the cheeks, nose and forehead), pustules and telangiectasia. Sometimes hyperplasia of the sebaceous glands and connective tissue of the nose is seen (rhinophyma).

The exact cause is unknown, however metronidazole cream has been shown to be effective, stepping up to oral antibiotics (i.e. tetracycline) if required. Steroids may worsen the rash.

Patients should be educated to protect themselves from excessive UV light exposure as this can exacerbate their rosacea.

Rosacea can resemble acne, so in exams remember these two key points:
- Acne is more common in younger patients and presents with comedones (blackheads and whiteheads).
- Rosacea has telangiectasia and no comedones.

Question 14

D *Pityriasis rosea*

It is an acute self-limiting rash characterized by scaly oval papules and plaques. Most patients have a single larger lesion, known as the 'herald patch', appear a few days before the rest of the rash manifests in a 'Christmas tree pattern'.

The cause of pityriasis rosea is unknown; however, it is suspected that the origin is infective, as a large number of patients report an upper respiratory tract infection in the preceding week.

It is a self-limiting condition (generally resolving within 3 months) and most patients are asymptomatic with it, although a quarter will suffer from pruritus, requiring antihistamines and topical steroids.

Question 15

1. B *Psoriasis*

Psoriasis is a chronic, non-infectious dermatosis. It is characterised by well-demarcated salmon coloured plaques, topped with silvery scales.

The plaques are typically considered to be found on extensor surfaces (knees and elbows) as opposed to the flexor surface distribution of eczema; however, there are many presentations of psoriasis (i.e. flexural psoriasis) and this is found on the flexor aspect, so don't be caught out.

The epidermis is thickened as the number of epidermal cells is increased sevenfold due to increased proliferation.

Causes include infections (i.e. streptococcal sore throat), drugs (beta-blockers, anti-malarials and lithium), cigarettes and alcohol, stress and the Koebner phenomenon (trauma to the skin, such as a cut or surgical scar, can set off psoriasis). Genetics are thought to play a substantial role in this disease, with 35% of patients having a family history of psoriasis.

2. D *Pethanol*

Pethanol is an analgesic drug and not used in the treatment of psoriasis. First-line treatment is with topical agents such as vitamin D analogues (calcipotriol), topical corticosteroids, coal tar preparations, retinoids and dithranol (an anti-mitotic).

Psoriasis can lead to erythroderma (when most of the skin on the body is affected by the disease) and in this case is a dermatological emergency requiring in-patient supportive treatment, as is explained later in this chapter.

Psoriasis may be complicated by arthropathy or become so severe it interferes with everyday life. Such cases may warrant systemic therapy in the form of methotrexate, ciclosporin and ultraviolet light treatment – UVB/PUVA (UVA light therapy + Psoralen, a drug that sensitizes the skin to the effects of UV light).

It is important to emphasize to patients that their rash is not infectious and health professionals must be particularly sensitive to the psychological impact that this unsightly rash has on the patient.

Question 16

Hereditary hemorrhagic telangiectasia (HHT), also known as Osler–Weber–Rendu disease, is an autosomal dominant disorder that leads to abnormal blood vessel formation. People with HHT lack capillaries in various areas of the body. This leads to arteries connecting directly with veins and so creating fragile vascular areas that can burst and bleed.

These abnormal vessels are called telangiectasias if small (such as on the skin surface, in the nose and stomach) and arteriovenous malformations when involving large vessels (i.e. in the liver, lung and brain). The main complications include:

- Internal bleeding – this may occur wherever these telangiectasias or arteriovenous malformations lie, thus leading to the possibility of haemorrhagic strokes, catastrophic rupture of vessels in the lungs and per rectum bleeding, leading to anaemia
- Pulmonary hypertension, due to arteriovenous malformations in the lungs
- Heart failure, due to high-flow liver arteriovenous malformations.

The skin lesions characteristically appear on the lips, nose and fingers (as seen in the images).

Treatment is directed to the areas where these abnormal vessels lie. Intervention is often surgical or involves embolisation by interventional radiologists. The important take-home message here is that these abnormal vessels are weak and more prone to rupture than a normal vessel. As a result-, these patients need careful monitoring and treatment before complications arise.

Question 17

This is a keratin (cutaneous) horn. Keratin horns typically arise on sun-exposed skin but can also be found in sun-protected areas. They occur more frequently in those > 60 years.

The horn is composed of compacted groups of large keratinocytes (not melanocytes). It is important to note that the hyperkeratosis resulting in horn formation occurs on the top of a hyperproliferative lesion. This lesion may well just be a simple wart, but in around 20% of cases it may be due to an underlying SCC.

Lesions that are large and grow rapidly (especially those with induration at the base) should be excised and sent for histopathological analysis. Smaller indolent lesions may be treated by curettage and cautery.

Beware using the word 'never' in exams – there are few certainties in medicine!

Question 18

1. B *Granuloma annulare*
The cause of this condition remains unknown and the vast majority of cases are seen in otherwise healthy people. Granuloma annulare's links to thyroid disease, AIDS and type 1 diabetes are unproven.

Roughly 50% of patients find that the rash resolves spontaneously within a couple of years, but unfortunately recurrence is relatively common.

2. C *No treatment required*
Patients are usually asymptomatic and often require little more than reassurance. Where treatment has been attempted, the success has been minimal and the scarring side-effects have outweighed the benefits. Intralesional steroids can be considered in more visible lesions, but repeated treatment is avoided due to the risk of cutaneous atrophy.

9 Ophthalmology[1]

Questions

Nick Muthiah and Michel Michaelides

Question 1

A 23-year-old woman presents to A&E complaining of grittiness, a mild discomfort and a burning sensation in her right eye. Her Snellen visual acuity is 6/6. The cornea shows superficial punctate staining with fluorescein. Her eyelid is shown below:

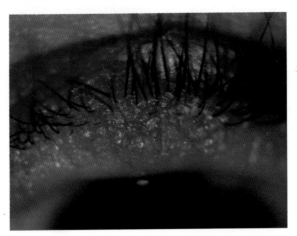

---

[1] All photographs in this chapter © Nick Muthiah

Clinical Data Interpretation for Medical Finals: Single Best Answer Questions, First Edition.
Edited by Philip Socrates Pastides and Parveen Jayia.
© 2012 Philip Socrates Pastides and Parveen Jayia. Published 2012 by John Wiley & Sons, Ltd.

What is the most likely diagnosis?
A. Foreign body
B. Stye
C. Allergic conjunctivitis
D. Blepharitis
E. Corneal abrasion

Question 2

A 70-year-old man presents to his GP with skin lesions over his right forehead and right upper lid. He had fever, malaise and headache preceding the rash. He also has tingling and a burning sensation over the right forehead. The skin lesions are shown below:

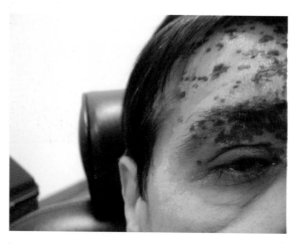

What is the most likely diagnosis?
A. Cellulitis
B. Trigeminal neuralgia
C. Herpes zoster ophthalmicus
D. Meningitis
E. Rosacea

Question 3

A 10-year-old boy attends his GP practice rubbing both his eyes vigorously and complaining of itching. His mother has been very concerned that this may affect his vision. She tells the GP that he is often like this during the spring/summer months. The only finding on examination is noted on everting his eyelids (shown below); his cornea is clear and the conjunctiva is mildly injected.

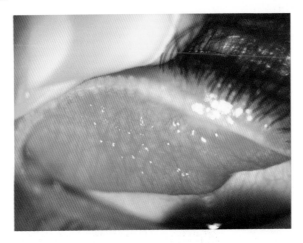

What is the diagnosis?
A. Corneal abrasion
B. Viral conjunctivitis
C. Allergic conjunctivitis
D. Foreign body
E. Chlamydial conjunctivitis

Question 4

A 35-year-old man presents to A&E with sore red eyes with a clear watery discharge. On examination he has bilateral preauricular lymphadenopathy. The photograph shows the conjunctival fornix. A week later he notices mild blurring of his vision. A photograph of the cornea is also shown.

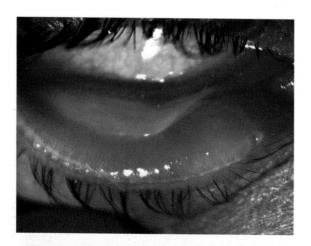

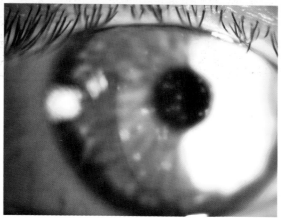

What is the most likely diagnosis?
A. Herpes simplex keratitis
B. Chlamydial keratoconjunctivitis
C. Allergic keratoconjunctivitis
D. Bacterial keratoconjunctivitis
E. Adenoviral keratoconjunctivitis

Question 5

A 34-year-old builder presents to A&E with his first episode of a painful right eye. It is watery and mildly photosensitive and he complains of a prickly sensation over the anterior surface of the eye. The junior doctor conducts an examination on the slit lamp with 2% fluorescein drops. The photograph is shown below:

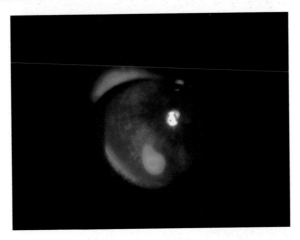

What is the diagnosis?

A. Foreign body
B. Recurrent corneal erosion
C. Dry eyes (keratoconjunctivitis sicca).
D. Corneal abrasion
E. Herpes simplex keratitis

Question 6

A teenager is brought in to A&E by his parents. He is complaining of severe pain in his left eye. It came on suddenly whilst he was grinding metal for his go-kart. A picture of his eye is shown:

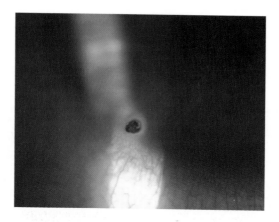

What does the picture show?

A. Corneal abrasion

B. Intraocular foreign body

C. Corneal foreign body

D. Conjunctival foreign body

E. Subtarsal foreign body

Question 7

A 30-year-old woman has shards of glass break in front of her when a pigeon flies into her window. She presents with a vision of 6/12 in her left eye. Her eye is injected, tearing and she is in pain. The photograph of her left eye is shown:

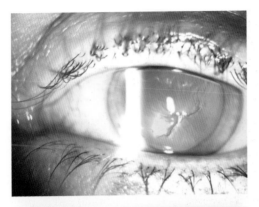

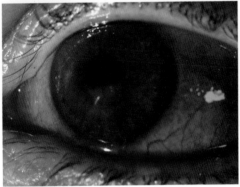

What should her management involve?

A. Diagnosis of a corneal abrasion, chloramphenicol ointment and pad for 24 hours

B. Diagnosis of a corneal foreign body, removal of this and chloramphenicol ointment

C. Diagnosis of a penetrating eye injury with full-thickness corneal laceration, referring patient urgently to the ophthalmic surgeons and protecting the eye with an eye shield

D. Diagnosis of a corneal ulcer, referring to ophthalmology and organising a corneal scrape in the meantime

E. Diagnosis of herpes simplex keratitis (dendrites), referring to ophthalmology and starting acyclovir eye ointment

Question 8

A 28-year-old female contact lens wearer presents to her GP with painful red eye, tearing and having noted her vision has decreased. She is mildly photosensitive. Upon further questioning she informs you that she has had similar episodes in the past and has just finished treatment with acyclovir for cold sores on her lips. On examination her Snellen acuity is 6/9. Her fluorescein stain is as shown below:

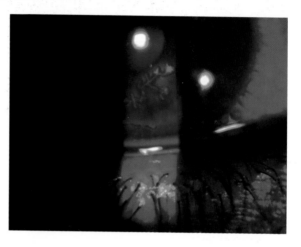

What is the diagnosis?
A. Fungal keratitis
B. Herpes simplex keratitis
C. Recurrent corneal erosion
D. Microbial keratitis (contact lens-related).
E. Corneal abrasion

Question 9

A 36-year-old with ankylosing spondylitis presents with a unilateral recurrent red and painful photophobic eye. He describes this as his third episode and informs you that his condition has settled previously with topical steroids and cyclopentolate drops. On examination the anterior segment of his eye is as shown:

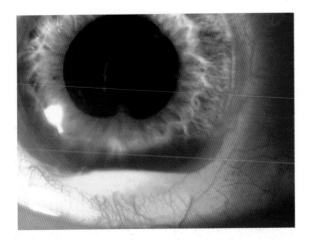

What is the diagnosis?

A. Herpetic zoster uveitis

B. Sarcoidosis

C. Behçet's disease

D. HLA-B27-associated acute anterior uveitis

E. Idiopathic anterior uveitis

Question 10

A 65-year-old male smoker with peripheral vascular disease is referred to the eye clinic by his GP due to decreased vision. It is currently 6/24 in both eyes. On fundus examination he is seen to have bilateral macular exudates in the form of a star. The patient also has attenuated arterioles (focal narrowing and sclerosis), arteriovenous nipping, retinal haemorrhages and cotton-wool spots.

What is the diagnosis?

A. Diabetic retinopathy

B. Central retinal vein occlusion

C. Hypertensive retinopathy

D. Central retinal artery occlusion

E. Age-related macular degeneration

Question 11

A 42-year-old woman with bilateral peripheral neuropathy and renal disease presents to A&E with a sudden decrease in the vision of her right eye and describes seeing a brown 'blob' in her right eye. Her right fundus photograph is seen below:

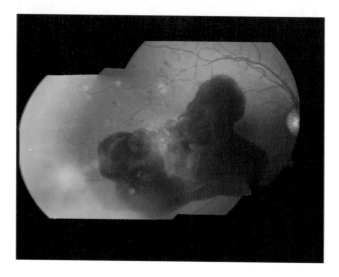

What is the most likely diagnosis?
A. Central retinal vein occlusion
B. Central retinal artery occlusion
C. Proliferative diabetic retinopathy
D. Retinitis pigmentosa
E. Rubella retinopathy

Question 12

A 67-year-old male with uncontrolled hypertension presented with sudden loss of vision in his right eye. He denied any ocular pain. His visual acuity was hand movement only. The right fundus photograph is shown:

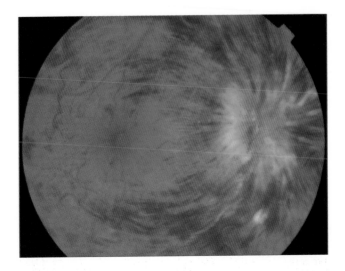

What is the most likely diagnosis?

A. Diabetic retinopathy

B. Hypertensive retinopathy

C. Central retinal vein occlusion

D. Central retinal artery occlusion

E. Vasculitis

Question 13

A 64-year-old smoker is referred by her optometrist due to mild blurring of central vision. She presents for a routine eye test. During her examination the findings are noted:

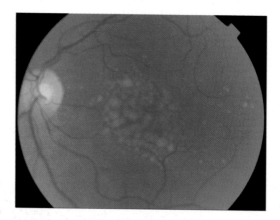

What is the most likely pathology?

A. Early dry age-related macular degeneration (drusen)

B. Wet macular degeneration

C. Atrophic age-related macular degeneration

D. Bull's eye maculopathy

E. Best macular dystrophy

Question 14

A 70-year-old woman presents to A&E with sudden distortion and blurring of central vision in her right eye. Her visual acuity is 6/18 in her right eye, the photograph of which is shown below:

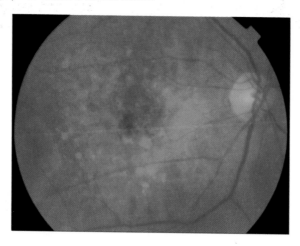

Following fundoscopy, what is the A&E doctor's diagnosis?

A. Wet age-related macular degeneration
B. Dry age-related macular degeneration
C. Atrophic macular degeneration
D. Diabetic maculopathy
E. Macular branch retinal vein occlusion

Question 15

A 48-year-old man who is visually asymptomatic is referred by his optometrist to your GP practice with the left fundus photograph as shown below. His visual acuity is 6/6 in both eyes.

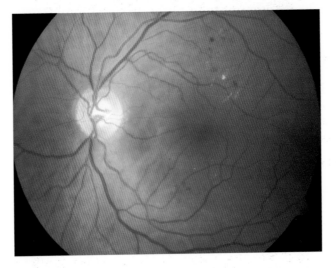

What is the diagnosis?

A. Hypertensive retinopathy with macular star exudates
B. Diabetic maculopathy
C. Dry macular degeneration (drusen)
D. Wet macular degeneration
E. Bull's eye maculopathy

Question 16

A 32-year-old woman with a history of rheumatoid arthritis presents to A&E with a painful red left eye. She is complaining of pain over the entire left orbit and also has pain on abduction of the left eye. Her vision is unaffected. Her left eye shown below:

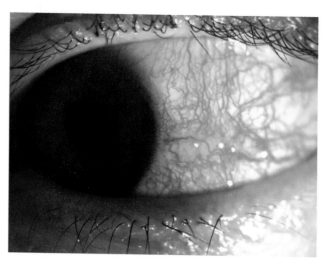

What is the diagnosis?
A. Conjunctivitis
B. Episcleritis
C. Scleritis
D. Uveitis
E. Trigeminal neuralgia

Question 17

A 10-year-old is brought to A&E by his mother. He has recently had an upper respiratory tract infection (URTI). He presents with swollen right upper and lower eyelids, and finds it difficult to open his eye. His conjunctiva is injected and chemosed. He has a right proptosis and reduced vision, as well as pain and diplopia in all positions of gaze. He is also noted to be pyrexial.

1. What is the diagnosis?
A. Pre-septal cellulitis
B. Orbital cellulitis
C. Allergic reaction
D. Scleritis
E. Retinoblastoma

2. What is the best course of management?

A. Oral antibiotics (co-amoxiclav) and discharge home

B. Admit, start IV antibiotics (ceftriaxone + metronidazole) and CT imaging

C. Admit, refer for CT imaging and await results before starting any treatment

D. Admit and await ophthalmology advice

E. Discharge home with ophthalmology and ENT outpatient appointments.

Question 18

A 28-year-old man who is highly myopic presents to A&E with sudden-onset flashing lights and floaters in the left eye. The junior doctor examining him notes that he has an inferonasal field defect in the left eye.

What is the likely diagnosis?

A. Temporal lobe stroke

B. Occipital lobe stroke

C. Migraine

D. Retinal detachment

E. Posterior vitreous detachment

Ophthalmology

Answers

Question 1

D Blepharitis

Blepharitis is a very common condition characterised by inflammation of the eyelid margin that causes non-specific ocular irritation and may be associated with staphylococcal infection of the base of the lashes (anterior blepharitis).

Non-infective blepharitis, also known as seborrhoeic anterior blepharitis, is associated with dysfunction of the glands of Zeis (modified sebaceous glands located at the base of the hair follicles which produce oily secretions). On examination you will see (as shown in the picture) lid margin erythema, crusting and scaling at the base of the eye lashes, and formation of collarettes around the bases of the lashes.

By contrast, posterior blepharitis is caused by dysfunction of the meibomian glands (sebaceous glands). These are located posterior to the lashes along the lid margin. The treatment in this patient will be regular lid hygiene (with warm compresses and lid hygiene). For suspected staphylococcal disease, chloramphenicol ointment twice a day to the lid margins for 2–3 weeks can be considered.

Question 2

C Herpes zoster ophthalmicus

Herpes zoster ophthalmicus, also known as ophthalmic shingles, usually presents many years after the primary infection. It is the reactivation of latent herpes zoster virus, which remains dormant in the dorsal root sensory ganglion. Reactivation occurs usually in the elderly but can occur in younger patients, especially if they are immunocompromised or immunosuppressed. Reactivation results in a localised cutaneous rash affecting a single dermatome; in this case it is the first division of the trigeminal nerve (ophthalmic distribution).

The presentation is a unilateral vesicular skin rash that does not cross the midline (respecting the dermatome). These vesicular lesions then crust and heal, often with residual scarring. An important sign to be aware of is Hutchinson's sign: this is when there are vesicles on the tip of the nose, signifying nasociliary nerve involvement and increasing the likelihood of ocular involvement.

A patient with this presentation should be started on oral acyclovir 800 mg five times a day for 7–10 days. This will accelerate healing, reduces neuralgia and the likelihood of ocular complications. The patient should be referred urgently for ophthalmological assessment.

Question 3

C *Allergic conjunctivitis*

Allergic conjunctivitis is often characterised by acute onset bilateral itching, lid oedema, conjunctival injection and chemosis. It is a very common type I hypersensitivity reaction that occurs during the hay fever season. Triggers can include pollen, grass, spores and pets.

Patients present with itching, tearing, redness and often a history of allergy. Symptoms are usually seasonal in nature, though it can be perennial.

Treatment is avoidance of the offending allergen, although this is usually difficult. Cool compresses, artificial tears and ideally a combined topical antihistamine and mast cell stabiliser eye drop such as olopatadine bd, or an over-the-counter mast cell stabiliser such as sodium cromoglycate drops qds.

Question 4

E *Adenoviral keratoconjunctivitis*

Adenoviral conjunctivitis is a common infection that is very contagious and almost always bilateral. The virus responsible is adenovirus and there are three typical presentations:

- Acute non-specific follicular conjunctivitis – produces red eye with irritation lid swelling and tearing; this will often resolve rapidly
- Epidemic keratoconjunctivitis involving serotypes 8 and 19, commonly seen in autumn and winter
- Pharyngoconjunctival fever is associated with serotype 3 and 7 and has systemic viral features.

It is important to ask patients about systemic features such as sore throat, fever and recent URTI. Contact history should be sought, as often the patient will have another close family member with similar symptoms. Conjunctival follicles are noted in the inferior fornix. Conjunctival pseudomembranes may also be noted in the fornices, as seen in the photograph.

Subepithelial corneal infiltrates (keratitis) can develop days to weeks after acute infection and this can significantly affect the visual acuity if it involves the visual axis and can also cause glare symptoms. This is shown in the second picture.

Treatment involves artificial tear drops and cool compresses. Antibiotics are not indicated unless there is suspicion of superimposed bacterial infection (unusual). In cases where there is involvement of the cornea, patients should be referred to an ophthalmologist for further management.

Question 5

D *Corneal abrasion*
Corneal abrasion is the commonest eye presentation in A&E. Often there is a history of a foreign body or mechanism by which the corneal epithelium has been breached. On the slit lamp you will see a corneal epithelial defect, which stains with fluorescein (as seen in the picture). There was no foreign body seen in the cornea in this case. Careful examination of the everted upper eyelid is also important to exclude a subtarsal foreign body.

Treatment is topical chloramphenicol ointment four times a day for 5–7 days. Some patients are more comfortable with a stat dose of chloramphenicol ointment and padding of the eye for 24 hours. Patients usually do not need review and can be discharged with advice to reattend if there is no improvement or worsening in symptoms by 36–48 hours. The patient should be reviewed in cases of large abrasions, i.e. > 50% of corneal involvement, due to the higher risk of infection.

Question 6

C *Corneal foreign body*
Junior doctors in A&E frequently see patients with corneal foreign bodies. Patients will complain of a foreign body sensation and ocular discomfort. Patients often also complain of photophobia and tearing. The history will often suggest the diagnosis. If there is potentially a high-velocity injury as sustained by striking or hammering metal or using power tools such as a jackhammer, this increases the risk of an intraocular foreign body and serious ocular injury.

In this case the picture shows a corneal metallic foreign body at the corneal limbus. The foreign body can be seen to be on the anterior corneal surface. There is no sign of a penetrating corneal wound.

Treatment involves removal of the foreign body using local anaesthetic and topical chloramphenicol eye drops qds for 5–7 days. It is also important to examine the anterior chamber for any intraocular foreign body or anterior chamber reaction and to check that the pupil is round and reactive. If the pupil is distorted, the anterior chamber is shallow or there is any evidence of lens injury, the patient should be referred for ophthalmological review to assess for a penetrating injury.

Question 7

C *Diagnosis of a penetrating eye injury with full-thickness corneal laceration, referring patient urgently to the ophthalmic surgeons and protecting the eye with an eye shield*

This woman has presented with a full-thickness corneal laceration sustained from the broken glass (top photograph). The bottom photograph shows a positive Seidel test. This test involves instilling fluorescein 2% drops. If there is aqueous leakage from the anterior chamber (as a consequence of a corneal laceration) the dark orange fluorescein 2% becomes diluted, turning bright green under cobalt blue light.

This confirms the globe is not intact and there is a penetrating eye injury. Other clues to a penetrating eye injury/ruptured globe are a shallow anterior chamber, a peaked/distorted pupil and iris or lens defect(s). These structures need to be assessed meticulously. Treatment is urgent referral to ophthalmology, protecting the eye with a cartella shield. It is helpful to arrange orbital X-rays to potentially localise any radio-opaque intraocular foreign body (IOFB).

Question 8

B *Herpes simplex keratitis*

Herpes simplex keratitis (HSK) is caused by HSV1 virus. It is a common condition that may occur as a primary infection in adults or children, but more commonly as a reactivation of a latent viral infection.

It is often recurrent HSK that presents to the GP or A&E and is often due to a recognisable trigger factor such as cold, stress or exposure to bright sunlight. Important features are single/multiple branching ulcerating epithelial lesions with raised irregular edges and bulb formation.

Prior to instilling the fluorescein 2% drops it is helpful to test for corneal sensation, as hypoaesthesia is often noted. Treatment is with topical acyclovir eye ointment five times a day for 2 weeks.

Question 9

D HLA-B27-associated acute anterior uveitis

All of the answers can cause uveitis. The commonest cause of acute anterior uveitis is idiopathic and HLA-B27-associated. HLA-B27 is positive in a number of systemic diseases, including ankylosing spondylitis, inflammatory bowel disease, Reiter's syndrome and psoriatic arthritis. These systemic diseases may all be associated with episodes of anterior uveitis.

In this photograph there is a hypopyon (inflammatory collection), keratic precipitates on the corneal endothelium and also noted is the irregular pupil due to posterior synechiae (adhesion of the iris to the lens capsule due to inflammation). The other hallmarks of acute anterior uveitis are perilimbal or circumcorneal injection and anterior chamber flare and cells. Patients should be referred to an ophthalmologist. It is inappropriate to start steroid eye drops without an ophthalmologist confirming the diagnosis.

Question 10

C Hypertensive retinopathy

The patient is a known arteriopath, and he has all the features of grade 3 hypertensive retinopathy. His vision is affected due to the exudates at the macula. His blood pressure needs to be checked and well controlled; he already has evidence of end-organ damage. He will need to be referred to the physicians. He is at a higher risk of myocardial infarction and stroke. The classification for hypertensive retinopathy is:

- Grade 1 – mild arteriolar narrowing
- Grade 2 – obvious focal arteriolar narrowing (due to spasm) and arterio-venous nipping
- Grade 3 – severe venous changes at arteriovenous crossings, flame-shaped haemorrhages, cotton-wool spots and hard exudates
- Grade 4 – disc swelling.

Question 11

C Proliferative diabetic retinopathy

This woman has presented with end-organ damage seen in patients with uncontrolled/undiagnosed diabetes mellitus. She has presented with retinal and vitreous haemorrhage secondary to bleeding of retinal new vessels. She described this as a brown 'blob'.

The proliferative diabetic retinopathy process is due to neovascularisation secondary to severe retinal ischaemia due to areas of retinal capillary closure. This results in increased retinal production of vascular endothelial growth factor (VEGF), which can lead to neovascularisation at the disc, retina and iris. This condition requires urgent pan-retinal laser photocoagulation.

These patients may also have other microvascular complications, such as renal disease and peripheral neuropathy. Importantly, randomised controlled trials have shown that tight glycaemic and blood pressure control considerably reduces the incidence and progression of retinopathy, nephropathy and neuropathy in type 1 and type 2 diabetes mellitus.

Question 12

C *Central retinal vein occlusion*

This patient has had a central retinal vein occlusion (CRVO). There are widespread retinal haemorrhages, gross unilateral disc swelling, dilated tortuous retinal veins, cotton-wool spots and macular oedema.

The commonest risk factors for this include age > 50 years and systemic diseases such as hypertension, diabetes and hyperlipidaemia. Glaucoma is another potential risk factor. If a patient is under the age of 50 then causes may include thrombophilia.

Investigations include blood pressure, full blood count, fasting blood glucose, and cholesterol. Patients need to be referred to physicians for further medical investigations. Ophthalmologists review these patients regularly to ensure they do not develop neovascular complications requiring treatment. There are also new treatments currently being evaluated that may be useful in managing macular oedema associated with CRVO, including intravitreal anti-VEGF injections and long-acting dexamethasone intravitreal implants.

Question 13

A *Early dry age-related macular degeneration (drusen)*

This lady has soft confluent drusen, which are a feature of age-related macular degeneration (ARMD). Patients initially are asymptomatic then gradually develop central vision problems. There is no history of sudden visual loss and no signs of haemorrhage or retinal oedema that may suggest wet age-related macular degeneration (neovascular ARMD).

There is a higher risk in white patients and smokers. Various genetic factors have been identified that increase the risk of ARMD, including variants in complement factor H and complement component 3 – consistent with an inflammatory aetiology. Patients are advised to stop smoking and supplement their diet with lutein and omega-3, which reduces their risk of progression and development of wet age-related macular degeneration.

Question 14

A *Wet age-related macular degeneration*

This picture shows widespread drusen (small yellow deposits lying deep to the retina). At the centre of the macula (fovea) there is an area of haemorrhage deep to the retina (subretinal haemorrhage). This is a result of a subretinal neovascular membrane, i.e. choroidal neovascularisation.

These patients should be referred urgently to the ophthalmologist for further management, which may include fundus fluorescein angiography and optical coherence tomography to confirm the presence of choroidal neovascularisation. Treatment involves injections of an anti-VEGF agent into the vitreous cavity.

Question 15

B *Diabetic maculopathy*

This patient's left fundus shows microaneurysms, dot haemorrhages and exudates at the left macula and they are approximately one disc diameter away from the fovea. The exudates have a discrete appearance, lying in the superficial layers of the retina, and are arranged in a circinate pattern, whereas drusen are deeper in the retina.

This is not hypertensive retinopathy as there are no vascular changes seen in the form of focal arteriolar narrowing or arteriovenous nipping. Bull's-eye maculopathy is a condition in which there is a concentric area of perifoveal hypopigmentation with central sparing in the early stages. It is seen in conditions such as Stargardt macular dystrophy and in drug toxicity (e.g. chloroquine and hydroxychloroquine).

In this patient treatment involves ensuring his risk factors are optimally controlled (blood sugar, blood pressure and cholesterol levels). Focal laser therapy is usually performed in patients with significant macula oedema. This patient has early diabetic maculopathy that at present does not require laser. He should be referred to the eye clinic.

Question 16

C *Scleritis*

This woman has anterior scleritis. This is an inflammatory disease affecting the sclera. This patient has an underlying systemic disease, rheumatoid arthritis. In approximately 50% of cases there is an association with a systemic disease.

Other diseases that can present with scleritis are Wegener's granulomatosis, polyarteritis nodosa and systemic lupus erythematosus. There is often a subacute onset of severe ocular pain that is worse with eye movement. There is also periocular pain that is deep, constant and boring which can affect sleep.

This patient requires urgent referral to an ophthalmologist. To help differentiate between episcleritis and scleritis, phenylephrine 2.5% eye drops can be instilled. This causes blanching of the superficial episcleral vessels but does not affect the deep scleral plexus.

Question 17

1. B *Orbital cellulitis*

This child has presented with a medical emergency: orbital cellulitis. It is a potentially life-threatening infection and may spread intracranially. The common source of infection is usually following an URTI, with the common microorganisms being staphylococci, streptococci and Haemophilus, although the latter is less common due to the Hib vaccine.

The possible sources of infection are paranasal sinuses, oropharynx, skin and, less commonly, trauma and a foreign body. The difference between pre-septal and orbital cellulitis is that, in orbital cellulitis, the severity and extent of ocular involvement are more noticeable in the form of proptosis, reduced and painful eye movement, conjunctival chemosis and reduced vision. By contrast, in pre-septal cellulitis there is gross lid oedema but none of the orbital signs mentioned above; in fact the eye is usually white. Patients are also systemically unwell with pyrexia with orbital cellulitis.

2. B *Admit, start IV antibiotics (ceftriaxone + metronidazole) and CT imaging*

Treatment involves urgent admission instituting high dose intravenous antibiotics without delay and fluid resuscitation (as the child in this case is pyrexial and potentially septic). CT scan is the imaging of choice to look for a subperiosteal abscess, collection within the orbit, as well as intra-cranial involvement.

Retinoblastoma is the commonest primary ocular malignancy occurring in children under 5 years old. The child will often have leucocoria (white pupillary reflex) and may have strabismus (squint) due to visual loss. It can very rarely cause secondary changes in the eye, such as orbital inflammation due to tumour necrosis (mimicking orbital cellulitis).

Question 18

D *Retinal detachment*
This man has risk factor for retinal detachment, as he is highly myopic (short-sighted). The significant warning signs for retinal detachment are an increase in floaters and flashing lights. The latter indicates traction on the retina, as the retina is being pulled during posterior vitreous detachment.

Visual field defects often occur once there is a retinal break and the retina has detached, and therefore it is important to refer patients as soon as they experience the initial warning sign. The commonest site for a retinal break/detachment is superiorly and this therefore accounts for an inferior field defect. The patient should be referred urgently to an ophthalmologist.

Patients with posterior vitreous detachment with no retinal breaks once reviewed by ophthalmologists can be safely discharged home with retinal detachment warning advice. Patients suffering from migraine will experience zig-zag lines and/or scintillating scotomata as their visual aura. Field tests are usually only abnormal during a migraine attack.

10 Evidence-based Medicine

Questions

Philip S. Pastides and Parveen Jayia

Question 1

Consider following numerical sequence:
11, 12, 53, 64, 87, 27, 21, 21, 53, 81, 3, 67, 53, 79, 7

1. What is the mode of this sequence?
A. 64
B. 3
C. 21
D. 53
E. 87

2. What is the approximate mean of this sequence?
A. 37
B. 40
C. 42
D. 44
E. 46

3. What is the median of this sequence?
A. 12
B. 21
C. 53
D. 67
E. 87

Clinical Data Interpretation for Medical Finals: Single Best Answer Questions, First Edition.
Edited by Philip Socrates Pastides and Parveen Jayia.
© 2012 Philip Socrates Pastides and Parveen Jayia. Published 2012 by John Wiley & Sons, Ltd.

Question 2

1. What is the primary assumption of a null hypothesis?
A. There is a real difference in the underlying population within the area of investigation.
B. There is no real difference in the underlying population within the area of investigation.
C. There could be a difference in the underlying population which is why the investigation is being carried out.
D. There is more than likely no difference in the underlying population within the area of investigation.
E. There is more than likely a real difference in the underlying population within the area of investigation.

2. Which of the following is true in relation to a type 1 error?
A. It is also known as a beta error.
B. It is seen when we conclude that there is a difference when actually there is no real difference.
C. It is seen when we conclude that there is no difference when actually there is a difference.
D. It is a false negative result.
E. It decreases as the *P* value increases.

3. Which one of the following is not true in relation to a type 2 error?
A. It is also known as a beta error.
B. It is seen when we conclude that there is no difference when there actually is a difference.
C. It Is a false-negative result.
D. It usually occurs because the sample size is too big.
E. It occurs if the null hypothesis is not rejected.

Question 3

A new blood test has been developed to detect condition X. It was tested on 100 people with the following results: 45 people tested positive for X and 45 actually had the condition; 10 people tested negative for the condition but were actually found to have the condition. The remainder who tested negative were found not to have the condition.

1. Which of the following is not a requirement of a screening test?

A. Cost-effectiveness
B. Effective treatment exists
C. Acceptable to the population
D. Non-invasive
E. Can be done in the community

2. What is the approximate sensitivity of the test?

A. 45%
B. 80%
C. 82%
D. 89%
E. 90%

3. What is the approximate specificity of the test?

A. 40%
B. 80%
C. 82%
D. 89%
E. 90%

Question 4

A new blood test has been developed to detect condition X. It was tested on 100 people: 50 people tested positive for X and 45 actually had the condition; 10 people tested negative for the condition but were actually found to have the condition. The remainder who tested negative were found not to have the condition.

1. What is the positive predictive value of the test?

A. 45%
B. 80%
C. 82%
D. 89%
E. 90%

2. What is the negative predictive value of the test?

A. 40%

B. 80%

C. 82%

D. 89%

E. 90%

Question 5

A new anti-migraine medication is being developed. It was tested on 40 patients who had suffered with at least two migraines in the last 2 months which were not relieved by existing anti-migraine medications. Twenty patients received the drug and 20 patients received a placebo. Neither patients nor medical staff knew which drug was being given to which group. They were followed up over the next 2 months to see whether or not they developed migraines. Two people receiving the drug developed a migraine within this time, whilst seven patients on the placebo drug developed a migraine within this time.

1. What type of study is this?

A. Single-blinded control trial

B. Double-blinded control trial

C. Open control trial

D. Cohort study

E. Experimental study

2. What is the absolute risk reduction with the new drug?

A. 10%

B. 25%

C. 35%

D. 65%

E. 90%

3. What is the number needed to treat?

A. 1

B. 2

C. 3

D. 4

E. 5

Question 6

Which one of the following statements about p value is correct?
A. It is the likelihood that a relationship under investigation is due to chance.
B. It is 100% accurate in determining a relationship.
C. It is statistically significant if less than 0.1.
D. It is statistically insignificant if less than 0.05.
E. It is an example of a non-parametric test.

Question 7

An odds ratio (OR) is used as a statistical value in which of the following studies?
A. Randomised control trial
B. Cohort study
C. Case–control study
D. Ecological study
E. Experimental study

Question 8

Which of the following statements is incorrect?
A. Point prevalence is the frequency of disease in a population at any given time.
B. Period prevalence is the frequency of disease in a population over a certain time period.
C. Incidence is the rate of occurrence of new disease in a population.
D. Incidence is the frequency of current disease in a population.
E. Standardised mortality ratio is the ratio of observed deaths to expected deaths in a given population.

Question 9

Which of the following statements is incorrect?
A. A cohort study identifies a group of people and follows them through time to see if a certain exposure causes a certain condition. This is then compared with a similar group of people not exposed to the exposure under investigation.
B. A case–control study compares a group of people with a certain condition with a group of people without that condition and looks back through time to evaluate any potential causative factors.
C. In an ecological study, the smallest unit of observation is a population or community. Ecological fallacy is a recognised error in this sort of study.
D. Vaccination is an example of primary prevention.
E. Screening is an example of tertiary prevention.

Question 10

Which of the following statements is incorrect?
A. In a single-blinded control trial, members of either the treating team or the patient group know which medication they are receiving.
B. Material published in a foreign language and excluded in a meta-analysis is an example of publication bias.
C. Confounding factors are factors outside of the search criteria that may affect results.
D. In a study with a 95% confidence interval of 1.32–1.49, $P < 0.05$ is statistically insignificant.
E. Randomisation is a method of reducing selection bias.

Question 11

A case–control study has been completed comparing 3000 female breast cancer suffers in the UK who have also has hip fractures. The study (see table below) states that more patients will have fractures whilst receiving oestrogen receptor antagonist (ORA).

	Received tamoxifen	Never prescribed ORA
Neck of femur fracture	516	296
No neck of femur fractures	984	1204
Total number of patients	1500	1500

What is the observed odds ratio?

A. 0.45
B. 0.62
C. 1
D. 2
E. 2.13

Question 12

A randomised control trial has just been published comparing the effect of a new antihypertensive medication, ZXA®, on Afro-Caribbeans. In the study the results have shown that patients who were given ZXA had better controlled blood pressure.

Which of the following statements best describes the hypothesis testing?

A. The null hypothesis is true (H_0).
B. One could always apply a one-tailed test to this study.
C. The null hypothesis has to be rejected.
D. The alternative hypothesis is true (H_1).
E. The alternative hypothesis is true.

Question 13

A recent study multi-centred, randomised control trial with a total recruitment of 25,000 has been published comparing the effects of a new bowel cancer drug. It states that there is a 45% reduction in 5-year mortality from bowel cancer in patients who have taken the new drug. The P-value was set before the study at $P < 0.05$. The study is asking you to reject the null hypothesis.

You reject the null hypothesis but a review article is published a month later which states that a significant number of patients were actually lost to follow-up and that there was in fact no difference in mortality between the two groups.

What type of error have you committed?

A. A type 1 error, as the alpha level not calculated
B. A type 1 error
C. A type 2 error
D. A type 1 and 2 error
E. No error at all

Question 14

You are asked to by your consultant to see if you can apply some statistics to a study he has been conducting, which is comparing exam results of module 2 following implementation of new teaching aid (e-modules). He wants to compare these results with the exam performance of the same students in module 1.

After analysing the data and establishing it is normally distributed, which one of the following would you apply?
A. Paired *t*-test
B. Wilcoxon signed-rank test
C. Unpaired *t*-test
D. Mann–Whitney *U*-test
E. One-way analysis of variance (ANOVA)

Question 15

A workforce analysis survey is being conducted at a major computer company. They are categorising the workforce into gender, age and ethnicity. The line manager is trying to decide which statistical test is best to apply.

Which one of the following should he choose?
A. One-way ANOVA
B. Chi-squared test
C. Paired *t*-test
D. Unpaired *t*-test
E. Wilcoxon signed rank test

Evidence-based Medicine

Answers

Question 1

1. D *53*
The first thing to do when faced with such a question is to carefully place the sequence in ascending numerical order:
3, 7, 11, 12, 21, 21, 27, 53, 53, 53, 64, 67, 79, 81, 87
The mode of a sequence is the number appearing most frequently within the sequence.

2. C *42*
The mean of a sequence is the sum of all the numbers in the sequence, divided by the number of numbers within that sequence.

3. C *53*
The median of a sequence is the number that appears in the middle of the sequence after it has been arranged in ascending numerical order

Question 2

1. B *There is no real difference in the underlying population within the area of investigation*
The primary assumption of a null hypothesis is that there is no real difference in the population under study and the study is set up to disprove this.

2. B *It is seen when we conclude that there is a difference when actually there is no real difference*
A type 1 error is also known as an alpha error. It is a false-positive result. The risk of a type 1 error decreases as the *P*-value decreases (i.e. it is less likely that it is due to chance).

3. D *It usually occurs because the sample size is too big*
A common occurrence of a type 2 error is that the sample size may be too small and hence give us the wrong impression

Question 3

For this type of question it may be easier to tabulate the information:

	Condition (+)ve	Condition (−)ve	Total
Test (+)ve	45 True positive (TP)	5 False positive (FP)	50
Test (−)ve	10 False negative (FN)	40 True negative (TN)	50
Total	55	50	

1. E *Non-invasive*
It also has to be as highly specific and sensitive to the disease under investigation as possible. It does not have to be done in the community, but this would be an added advantage as it would make it more accessible to the population.

2. C *82%*
Sensitivity is calculated as follows:

$$\frac{\text{Number who are both disease-positive and test positive (true positive)}}{\text{Total number of patients who are disease positive}}$$

or

$$TP/TP + FN$$

Now multiply by 100 to get the percentage.

3. D *89%*
Specificity is calculated as follows:

$$\frac{\text{Number who are both disease negative and test negative (true negative)}}{\text{Total number of patients who are disease negative}}$$

or

$$TN/FP + TN$$

Now multiply by 100 to get the percentage.

Question 4

For this type of question it may be easier to tabulate the information:

	Condition (+)ve	Condition (−)ve	Total
Test (+)ve	45	5	50
Test (−)ve	10	40	50
Total	55	50	

1. E 90%

The positive predictive value is the probability that a subject who tests positive for the condition actually has the condition. It is calculated as follows:

$$a/(a+b)$$

Multiply by 100 to get the percentage.

2. B 80%

The negative predictive value is the probability that a subject who tests negative for the condition actually does not have the condition. It is calculated as follows:

$$d/(c+d)$$

Multiply by 100 to get the percentage.

Question 5

For this type of question it may be easier to tabulate the information:

	Drug	Placebo	Total
Migraine (+)ve	2 (10%)	7 (35%)	9
Migraine (−)ve	18 (90%)	13 (65%)	31
Total	20	20	

1. B Double-blinded control trial

Double-blinded means that both parties are unsure as to which medication they are receiving. Single-blinded means one of the parties knows which drug is being given to which group, whilst in an open study, both parties know what they are receiving.

2. B 25%
Absolute risk reduction (ARR) is the decrease in risk of a new intervention compared with a control or pre-existing intervention. It is calculated as: (control event rate – experimental event rate). Even though it has 'reduction' in its name, it may actually be an increase.

3. D 4
The number needed to treat is the number of patients who need to be treated in order to prevent one additional bad outcome. It is calculated as (1/ARR).

Question 6

A *It is the likelihood that a relationship under investigation is due to chance*
A value of less than 0.05, by convention, is classified as statistically significant

Question 7

C *Case–control study*

Question 8

D *Incidence is the frequency of current disease in a population*
Incidence implies new disease frequency. All the definitions in the question should be known.

Question 9

E *Screening is an example of tertiary prevention*
Ecological fallacy is a recognised error in ecological studies. It assumes that all members of the population/community exhibit the same characteristics of the group at large.

Primary prevention is a method of preventing diseases, e.g. vaccination, while secondary prevention is a method of stopping early progression of a disease, e.g. screening. Tertiary prevention is a method of dealing with the effects of a disease, e.g. rehabilitation.

Question 10

D *In a study with a 95% confidence interval of 1.32–1.49, $P < 0.05$ is statistically insignificant*
A 95% confidence interval that does not cross 1 and has $P < 0.05$ is statistically significant.

Question 11

E 2.13

Odds ratio is calculated as follows:

$$\frac{\text{Odds of having fracture and not on tamoxifen } (516 \times 1204)}{\text{Odds of having fracture and taking tamoxifen } (984 \times 296)}$$

As patients are selected due to the fact that they already have a disease (breast cancer and hip fractures), it is not possible to estimate the absolute risk of disease using a case–control study.

Question 12

D The alternative hypothesis is true (H_1)

The null hypothesis is only true if the study showed that there was no reduction in blood pressure in either group (i.e. the new drug had no affect on patients' blood pressure). As there has been a reduction in blood pressure due to the medication, the alternative hypothesis is true. A one-tailed test means that you are expecting the results of the study to be in one direction, as already stated in the hypothesis.

Question 13

B A type 1 error

A type 1 error occurs when you reject the null hypothesis when actually it is true. Before any study, the maximum probability of making a type I error is calculated by the investigator and is the alpha (α) value. This is usually set at $P<0.05$, i.e. we will reject the null hypothesis if the P value is less than 0.05. A type 2 error occurs (denoted by beta, β) when we accept the null hypothesis when actually a difference exists. The chance of this occurring is controlled by the power of the study. The higher the power of the study, the less likely it is that this will occur.

Question 14

A Paired t-test

Paired *t*-test is applied to parametric data that are normally distributed and are related to each other. The data here are related to each other as they are following the same individuals. The Wilcoxon signed-rank test is for related groups of data that are not normally distributed. The Mann–Whitney *U*-test can be used for non-parametric data that are not related to each other. ANOVA is applied to data that are from more than two unrelated groups.

Question 15

B *Chi-squared test*

The data that will be generated will be categorical data, meaning each individual either possess a characteristic or not (i.e. they are male or female). As we are analysing more than one categorical function, we will use the chi-squared test. The other tests mentioned in the question are only applied to numerical data.

Appendix A: How to Interpret an ECG

Interpretation of ECG is one of the key tasks encountered in clinical practice. Most emergencies in cardiology can be recognised by ECG and hence it is vital that ECGs are accurately assessed. In the first few years of clinical practice, one has to employ methodical steps to interpret ECGs in order to ensure that essential findings are not missed. The following steps will help to in making accurate assessments.

1. Rate, rhythm and axis deviation

It is always helpful to start with these.

Rate
Normal heart rate is in the range 60–100 beats/min. A lower heart rate could be due to sinus bradycardia and heart blocks (Mobitz type 2 and complete heart block). A faster heart rate could be due to sinus tachycardia, atrial or ventricular tachyarrhythmias. It could also be due to atrioventricular (AV) nodal re-entry tachycardias.

Rhythm
The commonest rhythm disturbances encountered in clinical practice are atrial fibrillation, supraventricular and ventricular ectopics. Those less commonly encountered are atrial flutter, atrial tachycardia, AV nodal re-entry tachycardias and ventricular tachycardia.

Axis deviation
Axis deviation indicates a shift in the electrical and/or mechanical axis of the cardia. For example, left axis deviation could be encountered in individuals with left ventricular enlargements or left anterior hemi-block. Right axis deviation is usually seen in individuals with right ventricular hypertrophy or left posterior hemi-block.

Clinical Data Interpretation for Medical Finals: Single Best Answer Questions, First Edition.
Edited by Philip Socrates Pastides and Parveen Jayia.
© 2012 Philip Socrates Pastides and Parveen Jayia. Published 2012 by John Wiley & Sons, Ltd.

2. Individual waves and complexes

P wave

P-wave abnormalities reflect structural changes in the atrium. For example, P-mitrale (bifid P waves) indicates left atrial enlargement and P-pulmonale (tall P waves) indicates right atrial enlargement.

QRS complex

A prolonged QRS complex indicates a block in the right or left bundle. A right bundle branch block is characterised by the presence of a tall and prolonged R wave in lead V1. A left bundle branch block is characterised by the presence of a deep and broadened S wave in lead V1 and a prolonged R wave in lead V5–V6.

The amplitude of the QRS complex across the pre-cordial leads may also indicate left or right ventricular hypertrophy.

ST segment and T wave

These provide important information during myocardial ischaemia or infarction. Changes during ischaemia include T-wave inversion and/or ST-segment depression. ST-segment elevation always denotes impending ischaemia.

QT interval

This reflects ventricular repolarisation. A prolonged QT interval could be due to either acquired causes, such as electrolytes disturbances (low potassium, magnesium or calcium), or QT-prolonging drugs (erythromycin, antihistamines, amitryptilline, chlorpromazine, sotalol, amiodarone, antifungals). In a small proportion of individuals it is congenital as a result of mutations in the sodium or potassium channels of cardiac myocytes.

Appendix B: How to Interpret a Chest Radiograph

Books have been written about how to interpret a chest radiograph. Having a systematic approach, such as the one outlined in this appendix, will reduce the likelihood of you missing any abnormalities. A normal chest radiograph is shown below:

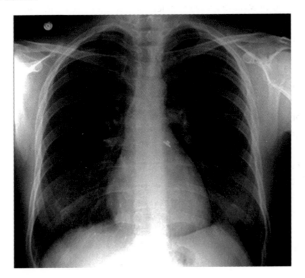

Check the following:
1. What the investigation is showing ('This is a plain chest radiograph') followed by whether it is posteroanterior (PA) or anteroposterior (AP)
2. Patient demographics (name of patient, age, date and time of investigation)
3. Any obvious abnormalities
4. Starting centrally, start with the trachea (midline?)

Clinical Data Interpretation for Medical Finals: Single Best Answer Questions, First Edition.
Edited by Philip Socrates Pastides and Parveen Jayia.
© 2012 Philip Socrates Pastides and Parveen Jayia. Published 2012 by John Wiley & Sons, Ltd.

5. Heart (including behind the heart) and mediastinal contours (including size of hila)
6. Cardiophrenic angles
7. Costophrenic angles
8. Below the diaphragm
9. Lung fields (in particular, check the apices carefully)
10. Ribs (six anterior ribs or 10 posterior ribs are normal; more than this suggests hyperexpansion)
11. Other bones (especially clavicles, scapulae, humera) and soft tissues (surgical emphysema)
12. Additional points (i.e. foreign objects, endotracheal tubes, nasogastric tubes, pacemakers, ECG/cardiac monitor stickers)

Appendix C: How to Interpret an Arterial Blood Gas

Arterial blood gases (ABGs) are a very useful investigation in many patients, especially those who are very unwell.

Obtaining an ABG is half the battle – they are only useful if interpreted correctly and acted upon appropriately. Like many things in medicine, ABGs are all about having a systematic interpretation. Below we outline a system for interpreting ABGs which you can choose to adopt. However, you may already have your own system that covers the same points.

1. pH – Is the patient acidaemic (pH < 7.35) or alkalaemic (pH > 7.45)?
2. PO2 – On room air (21%) the patient should have a PO2 of around 10–13kPa. This normal can be slightly lower in an elderly patient.
   a. This needs to be interpreted in the context of the inspired oxygen concentration.
3. Saturations (SO_2) – Normally greater than 94%
   a. Can vary if the patient has chronic obstructive pulmonary disease – or any other cause of respiratory disease/pulmonary oedema etc.!
4. PCO_2 – Normally in the range 4.5–6 kPa – adjusted by the lungs.
   a. If this is raised then it would cause an acidaemia on its own. The only cause of hypercapnia is hypoventilation. This is due to a decreased minute ventilation, i.e. respiratory rate × tidal volumes, caused by: a reduced respiratory rate (such as opiate overdose) or low tidal volume [such as with muscle weakness, chronic obstructive pulmonary disease (COPD)]
   b. If PCO_2 is low then it would cause an alkalaemia on its own. This is due to an increased minute ventilation, generally secondary to an increased respiratory rate, e.g. acute exacerbation of asthma, psychogenic hyperventilation.
   c. It may be abnormal if compensating for a metabolic defect.

Clinical Data Interpretation for Medical Finals: Single Best Answer Questions, First Edition.
Edited by Philip Socrates Pastides and Parveen Jayia.
© 2012 Philip Socrates Pastides and Parveen Jayia. Published 2012 by John Wiley & Sons, Ltd.

5. HCO_3 – Normally in the range 22–28 kPa – adjusted by the kidneys.
   a. If this is raised then it would cause an alkalaemia on its own.
   b. If this is low then it would cause an acidaemia on its own.
   c. It may be abnormal due to compensation for a respiratory defect.
6. Base excess – Normally between −2 and +2 mmol/L
   a. Generally deranged in the same direction as the bicarbonate concentration.
7. Lactate – Normally below 1.6 mmol/L.
   a. Deranged in any cause of organ hypoperfusion, e.g. systemic hypotension.
8. Glucose – 4–8 mmol/L.
9. Other electrolytes
   a. e.g. Sodium, potassium, chloride
10. Interpretation
    a. Can be split into respiratory or metabolic and acidosis or alkalaosis as the primary cause. Acideamia and alkalaemia refer to the pH.
    b. If the PCO_2 is abnormal, check the bicarbonate – e.g. if the CO_2 and bicarbonate are raised then this would (usually) be metabolic compensation.

Appendix D: How to Interpret an Abdominal Radiograph

System for reviewing film

1. Technical factors
Check the name, age and sex of the patient. Ensure the side marker is accurate. Technical factors such as rotation and projection do not make a significant impact on the interpretation. Confirm that the whole of the abdomen is covered on the film, from diaphragm to groin/proximal femur.

2. Solid organs
Accurate delineation of the solid organs of the abdomen is usually not possible. The outline of the right lobe of liver, kidneys and bladder may be seen in some patients. In the majority of cases, it is possible to clearly outline the border of the psoas muscle bilaterally. The absence of this outline raises the possibility of retroperitoneal pathologies.

3. Hollow organs (bowel)
It is normal to see gas within the stomach, two to three loops of small bowel, colon and the rectum.

4. Bones
Assess the vertebrae, pelvic bones, ribs and joint spaces.

5. Abnormal densities/opacities
Look for foci of abnormal density/opacities in the abdomen, especially along the renal tract. The majority of the renal calculi are visible on an abdominal X-ray. In many centres, non-contrast CT of the renal tract is being used for detection of renal calculi in place of abdominal X-ray.

6. Review areas
These are areas that are often missed on an abdominal X-ray. Check the lung bases, aorta and groins/hernial orifices.

Clinical Data Interpretation for Medical Finals: Single Best Answer Questions, First Edition.
Edited by Philip Socrates Pastides and Parveen Jayia.
© 2012 Philip Socrates Pastides and Parveen Jayia. Published 2012 by John Wiley & Sons, Ltd.

Abnormalities

A thorough knowledge of the normal appearances of the structures listed above will enable identification of abnormalities. Abnormalities include structures being too large, too small or absent. Displacement, abnormal shape or density of structures should be identified. Opacities or areas of abnormal density may be present on the film.

The main densities on a plain radiograph are as follows:

- Metallic – bright white
- Bone/calcium – white
- Soft tissue/fluid – grey
- Fat – dark grey
- Gas – black

Common or important abnormalities

Solid organs

If the liver is significantly enlarged, this may be seen on abdominal X-ray. An abnormal outline of the kidneys due to a structural abnormality or tumour may be seen. Enlargement/absence of kidneys may also be identified. Inability to visualise the border of psoas could represent serious pathology (e.g. retroperitoneal haemorrhage) but could also bee due to benign factors (e.g. overlying gas or abdominal fat).

Hollow organs

Dilated bowel could represent mechanical obstruction, ileus, pseudo-obstruction or other rarer pathology. The colon is considered dilated if it measures more than 5.5 cm in diameter and the caecum over 9 cm. Small bowel distension > 2–2.5 cm is considered abnormal.

Large bowel tends to be more peripheral than small bowel, contains faeces unlike small bowel and tends to contain more gas. Haustrations in the colon do not cross the entire width of the colon and tend to be broader and more widely spaced compared with the valvulae conniventes in small bowel, which cross the entire small bowel, are narrower and closer to each other.

When the colon is inflamed (e.g. inflammatory bowel disease, colitis) the bowel wall mucosa becomes oedematous and can lead to the appearance of 'thumbprinting'.

Bones

Primary or metastatic bone tumours lead to destruction or abnormal morphology of bones. Traumatic or osteoporotic fractures may also be identified. Assessing joint spaces enables identification of degenerative change.

Calcification

Renal calculi can be identified in the renal tract/bladder as high-density, calcific opacities. Try to differentiate these from phleboliths in the pelvis which have a smoother border, a lucent centre (not always seen) and are not projected over the track of the renal tract.

Gallstones may be identified as calcific opacities over the right upper quadrant, but only 10% of gallstones are visible on abdominal X-ray.

Look for vascular calcification. This is particularly important in identifying abdominal aortic aneurysms – a high index of suspicion could lead to picking up a calicifed aortic aneurysm.

Pneumoperitoneum

Perforation of a viscus leads to free intraperitoneal air. Abdominal X-ray is less sensitive than chest X-ray in picking up this abnormality, but visualising air on both sides of the bowel wall ('Rigler's sign') is indicative of free gas. Gas outlining the falciform ligament is also consistent with free intraperitoneal air. Free subdiaphragmatic air may also be seen on abdominal X-ray, in keeping with pneumoperitoneum.

Apparent free subdiaphragmatic air is seen when the colon is interposed between the liver and diaphragm (Chilaiditi's syndrome) simulating pneumoperitoneum – it is important to distinguish this from a true perforation.

Foreign objects

Foreign bodies may be seen on abdominal X-ray, e.g. due to ingestion/ insertion by patient or secondary to trauma.

Remember, a systematic approach, understanding of normal appearances and accurate description of abnormalities will enable diagnosis of pathology.

Appendix E: How to Interpret a CT Head

Computed tomography of head (CTH) is becoming one of the most common imaging investigations performed in A&E and medical emergency units. In current UK practice, the scan is usually accompanied by a report from a radiologist. Therefore, junior doctors are not expected to report on the scan.

In this section we will briefly outline a systematic approach and outline findings in most common conditions.

Images are acquired in the scanner with patients lying on their back (supine). The use of IV contrast is reserved for specific clinic indications, including possible meningitis, possible abscess and possible malignancy.

First of all, ensure the patient details, date of scan and clinical information are correct. The normal density of the brain is grey, cerebrospinal fluid (CSF) is black and bone is white. In a normal patient, it should be possible to clearly identify the sulci and gyri of the brain and there should not be any high density within the brain parenchyma. The ventricles contain dark-coloured CSF but it is also common to see some calcification within the lateral ventricles. The size of the ventricles, especially the temporal horn of the lateral ventricle, helps in determining the presence or absence of hydrocephalus. It is important to ascertain that there is no shift of the midline as this may indicate significant pathology. The cranial bones should also be looked at closely in bone windows to exclude fractures.

Pathologies

These can be broadly differentiated into: infarct, haemorrhage, mass.

Infarct

The density of the infarcted brain varies depending on the duration of infarct. In hyperacute stages, brain parenchyma may be normal in appearance and it may be possible to see an area of hyperdensity within the middle cerebral artery. In acute to subacute stages, the density of the infarcted brain lowers (more dark), and in the chronic stage it attains the same signal as that of the CSF (black). The areas of abnormal density tend to follow the vascular distribution and are usually unilateral.

Clinical Data Interpretation for Medical Finals: Single Best Answer Questions, First Edition.
Edited by Philip Socrates Pastides and Parveen Jayia.
© 2012 Philip Socrates Pastides and Parveen Jayia. Published 2012 by John Wiley & Sons, Ltd.

Haemorrhage

Acute haemorrhage has a higher density (white) than the brain matter. Four types of haemorrhage can be encountered:

- Extradural haemorrhage – this is a medical emergency and requires urgent neurosurgical attention. There is usually a history of trauma with a fracture of the skull. The haemorrhage is extra-axial (extra-parenchymal), hugs the outer surface of the brain and has a convex inner border. The density of the blood is bright.
- Subdural haemorrhage – this is usually seen in elderly patients and there may or may not be a history of trauma or a skull fracture. This also needs requires discussion/referral to the neurosurgical team. This is also an extra-axial haemorrhage but has a 'concave' inner border. The density of the blood can be mixed (both bright and dark), as the clinical presentation may not be acute.
- Intra-parenchymal – this is an intra-axial haemorrhage and is seen as an area of increased density within the brain matter. Common causes for this include hypertension, trauma and malignancy.
- Subarachnoid haemorrhage – patients usually present with a history of severe headache with photophobia. High-density blood can be seen within the subarachnoid space along the vessels, sulci/gyri and within the ventricles.

Mass

Adult intracranial masses are metastases, primary malignancy or benign tumours. They may be inconspicuous in a plain CTH without contrast and MRI of the brain is usually required to further characterise these masses. The density of the masses can vary significantly, with some of the primary/secondary lesions demonstrating calcification (bright) or necrosis (dark). A tumour is usually associated with a peripheral area of low density due to ongoing oedema. A tumour may also have significant mass effect leading to obstruction/dilatation of the ventricles (hydrocephalus) and or herniation of the brain to the contralateral side (shift of midline).